KT-104-619

10 Signs You're Not Dressing for Success

1. **You dress for the job you have.** If you look like all the other employees at your level, that's how you'll continued to be seen. Dress for the position you want, however, and people are more likely to believe that you're qualified to do it.

2. **Your shoes aren't polished and in good repair.** Those in charge put a lot of stock in the state of an employee's— or perspective employee's—shoes. (For some, it ranks right up there with a firm handshake.) Your shoes should always be shiny and well-heeled.

3. **You dress the same way you did in college.** The corporate world is a long way from the campus, especially in terms of what's considered acceptable attire. Many offices won't tolerate jeans and T-shirts, no matter how casual the environment. Now's the time to graduate to some more grown-up clothes.

4. **You have lots of low-quality clothing.** Poorly constructed clothing can put the kibosh on a professional image. Better to have less clothing of a higher quality.

5. **You always shop at the 11th hour.** Unless you shop best under pressure, you're probably buying clothing that doesn't really fit the bill, in one significant way or another. To be sure your wardrobe is sending the right message, plan ahead.

6. **Most of your clothes are stained, wrinkled, or missing buttons.** Remember that one little ding will spoil the perfect paint job.

7. **You follow fashion trends closely.** It's annoying, but true: Wearing what's "hot," especially if it's informal or otherwise inappropriate for work, can really bother some bosses. Better to stick with classic styles that flatter your physique, and express you fashion individuality after hours and on weekends.

8. **The only casual clothes you own are sweats and jeans.** In this day of casual Fridays, you need to be able to dress the part without sacrificing your professionalism.

9. **It's been three months since your last haircut.** You can't discount the importance of good grooming to your overall appearance. Shaggy hair, dirty nails, and poor personal hygiene will undermine your chances as surely as a missed deadline or a bad attitude.

10. **You can't pull an interview or meeting-appropriate outfit together in a hurry.** When opportunity knocks, you need to be ready—a problem if nothing in your closet quite mixes or matches with anything else. At the very least, have on hand one ensemble that makes you feel comfortable and confident.

alpha
books

10 Things Every Well-Dressed Person Must Own

1. A lint brush
2. A sewing kit
3. An iron and ironing board
4. A full-length mirror
5. A good pen
6. An elegant (though not necessarily expensive!) watch
7. Shoe polish
8. A wool blazer
9. A quality umbrella
10. A copy of *The Complete Idiot's Guide to Successful Dressing*

10 Keys to Successful Dressing

1. Recognize that you have less than 10 seconds to make a good impression.
2. Know that what you wear influences others and can at least make you appear to be more confident and in control.
3. Focus on being appropriately dressed—every day.
4. Plan ahead; don't "wing it."
5. Avoid attire that makes others feel uncomfortable. You want to stand out for your performance, not your clothes.
6. Develop a consistent style of dress that takes into account your physical assets and flaws.
7. Spend enough to make the grade. It's worth it to splurge on one or two great outfits that make you feel invulnerable.
8. Play it safe. When in doubt, dress conservatively.
9. Take cues from your superiors.
10. Sweat the small stuff. Attention to detail is a virtue that employers look for in an employee's work and wardrobe.

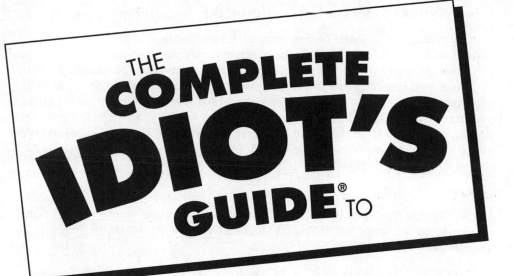

THE COMPLETE IDIOT'S GUIDE® TO

Successful Dressing

by Karyn Repinski

alpha books

A Division of Macmillan General Reference
1633 Broadway, New York, NY 10019-6785

Copyright © 1999 by Karyn Repinski

All rights reserved. No part of this book shall be reproduced, stored in a retrieval system, or transmitted by any means, electronic, mechanical, photocopying, recording, or otherwise, without written permission from the publisher. No patent liability is assumed with respect to the use of the information contained herein. Although every precaution has been taken in the preparation of this book, the publisher and author assume no responsibility for errors or omissions. Neither is any liability assumed for damages resulting from the use of information contained herein. For information, address Alpha Books, 1633 Broadway, 7th Floor, New York, NY 10019-6785.

THE COMPLETE IDIOT'S GUIDE TO & Design is a registered trademark of Prentice-Hall, Inc.

Macmillan Publishing books may be purchased for business or sales promotional use. For information please write: Special Markets Department, Macmillan Publishing USA, 1633 Broadway, New York, NY 10019.

International Standard Book Number: 0-02-862729-6
Library of Congress Catalog Card Number: 98-89725

01 00 99   8 7 6 5 4 3 2 1

Interpretation of the printing code: the rightmost number of the first series of numbers is the year of the book's printing; the rightmost number of the second series of numbers is the number of the book's printing. For example, a printing code of 99-1 shows that the first printing occurred in 1999.

Printed in the United States of America

Note: This publication contains the opinions and ideas of its author. It is intended to provide helpful and informative material on the subject matter covered. It is sold with the understanding that the author and publisher are not engaged in rendering professional services in the book. If the reader requires personal assistance or advice, a competent professional should be consulted.

The author and publisher specifically disclaim any responsibility for any liability, loss or risk, personal or otherwise, which is incurred as a consequence, directly or indirectly, of the use and application of any of the contents of this book.

Alpha Development Team

Publisher
Kathy Nebenhaus

Editorial Director
Gary M. Krebs

Managing Editor
Bob Shuman

Marketing Brand Manager
Felice Primeau

Editor
Jessica Faust

Development Editors
Phil Kitchel
Amy Zavatto

Production Team

Development Editor
Carol Hupping

Production Editor
Donna Wright

Copy Editor
June Waldman

Cover Designer
Mike Freeland

Photo Editor
Richard H. Fox

Photography
Roch Craford

Illustrator
George McKeon

Designers
Scott Cook and Amy Adams of DesignLab

Indexer
John Jefferson

Layout/Proofreading
Carrie Allen
Eric Brinkman
Ellen Considine

Contents at a Glance

Contents

8 The Basic Components 81

9 Accessories: Special Effects 103

Foreword

You only have one chance to make a first impression, and Karyn Repinski shows you how to make certain it's a good one. Her wonderful fashion sense and wise advice will serve you and your wardrobe well on the job, every day—whether you're prepping for an important meeting or a job interview, packing for a trip, or getting ready for an appearance on national television.

If you want to be seen as a winner at work, you've got to dress the part, be it conservative corporate, creative, casual, or anything in between. Let *The Complete Idiot's Guide to Successful Dressing* be your savvy guide on what to wear and when to wear it.

Saralee Terry Woods
A staffing industry consultant and author of *Executive Temping—A Guide for Professionals*, John Wiley & Sons, Inc., 1998.

Introduction

The first time I ever really experienced the consequences of dressing inappropriately was when I was a junior in college taking a class in business communications. For our last assignment, which counted for something like a third of our grade, we had to make group presentations on a topic I have since forgotten. What I remember clearly, however, was the weight the teacher assigned to how the group was dressed.

Though she didn't elaborate much, she left little doubt that she was expecting us to look like professional businessmen and businesswomen. Considering that it was 1981, the height of the dress-for-success period, which prescribed conservative suits (with skirts for women) as the requisite get-ahead garb, I figured that was what we would all be wearing.

Because I wanted to be sure to get an A in this class, I mentioned the importance of looking sharp to my group when we met the night before the presentation. To me, dressing the part was the easiest aspect of the whole assignment, and there didn't seem to be any reason to lose points over it. In response to my reminder, everyone agreed to be dressed appropriately.

Well, I'm sure you're way ahead of me here, having guessed that most of the team wasn't suited up for business after all. One woman wore a dinner suit, the kind with lace around the lapels, while the other wore gray polyester pants and a red blouse. One of the guys had on corduroy jeans (they were new, he pointed out) and was conspicuously tieless under his V-neck sweater.

What the heck was going on, I wondered? Were they purposely trying to sabotage our chance for success? Didn't they know what constituted professional attire? As it turned out, they didn't. And you know what? As is evident in office building corridors across the country, the situation hasn't changed much. Especially in this era of relaxing dress codes, confusion still reigns when it comes to dressing appropriately for work—a troubling trend, considering the stakes. Indeed, knowing the weight those in the position of hiring place on appearance, not dressing up to snuff could be tantamount to professional suicide. Even with the IQ of Einstein, if you looked as scruffy as he often did, your lack of fashion savvy could sink you on the employment front.

(For those of you wondering about my grade, I still managed to pull off an A. I've always wondered, if my professor took pity on me, or if she was just a softie at heart.)

How to Use This Book

Our goal here—that is, mine in writing this book and yours in reading it—is to arm you with the knowledge you need to project a winning impression. To lead you in an organized fashion through all the relevant information, this book is arranged in six parts.

Part 1, Dress to Impress, This is where you'll learn about the crucial role clothing plays on the job, the growing trend toward casual dressing, and the importance of dressing like a team player.

Part 2, The Educated Consumer, It's not about how much money you spend on your work wardrobe, but about knowing the difference between a bad investment (a shoddy suit) and a good one (a does-it-come-in-other-colors-too cashmere sweater). These chapters will help make you a much more savvy shopper.

Part 3, Building a Wardrobe, What in your closet works, and what doesn't? What clothing and accessories are best suited to you and your work style? How can you create a wardrobe that really coordinates, and then get the most out of it? What more could you ask from five chapters?

Part 4, Special Performances, The information in these three chapters may not yet be relevant to you. But when you get the call ("We'd love to talk with you about our job opening," "...meet with you about handling our account," "...discuss the issue over lunch," "...have you as a speaker at our meeting"), you'll have it at your fingertips.

Part 5, Special Conditions, Travel. Rain and Snow. Heat. A baby! The four chapters here coach you on how to deal with special situations.

Part 6, Survival Skills, First, there's the matter of grooming and personal hygiene, followed by the subject of camouflaging figure flaws. Next up is the skinny on those thorny issues that no one ever discusses until the damage is already done: hem length, beards, and cultural expression. A primer on clothing care and shopping strategies comes next, followed by advice for the cash-strapped and those in need of more help.

Off the Cuff

In addition to advice, anecdotes, explanations, and examples, you'll see at least one of these four boxes on almost every page of the book. Be sure to read them because they're chock-full of practical pointers and entertaining extras.

The Fashion Police

The information in these boxes will alert you to potential problems and prevent you from making career-sabotaging missteps.

Dollars & Sense

These boxes contain tips on how to minimize the expense of a working wardrobe.

Fashion Footnote

Here you'll find definitions, facts, and other nuggets of interesting and useful information.

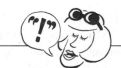

Quote . . . Unquote

Amusing observations, uproarious one-liners, and true words of sartorial wisdom can be found here.

Acknowledgments

The name on the cover of this book may be mine, but I couldn't have completed this project without lots of help and support from a number of people—most notably, my husband and collaborator, Roch Craford; my sister, Kimm Repinski; my good friends (who, coincidentally, also happen to be great writers) Audrey "A.J." Hanley and Victoria Clayton; and my parents.

My sincere thanks is also extended to the following individuals and colleagues for generously sharing with me their valuable insights on this subject: Marie Amadio, Valeri Audino, Lynn Bradach, Karen Bressler, Mike Casey, Mari Connolly, Steve Connolly, Mary Margaret Craford, Mike Craford, Lucy Cutting, Mary Lou DiNardo, Paula Dorf, Mary Early, Teresa Flack, Jody Kozlow Gardner, Jane Scott Grant, Linda Haneborg, Linda Hudak, Janis Jibrin, Danny Kraus, Emily Lyons, Barbara Manning, Karpagam Maran, Kevin McCauliffe, Rebecca McCauliffe, Marnie McLaughlin, Jayne Morehouse, Eric Morgan, Paula Musely, Joyce Newman, Tricia O'Connor, Angela O'Mara, Kendall Ong, Shannon O'Rourke, Sonja Popp, Maura Rhodes, Jackie Riley, Julie Rosch, Helene Rosenzweig, M.D., Maureen Ryan, Teresa Scanlon, Cheri Serota, Harris Shephard, Suzanne Simons, William Sullivan, Kerry Tice, Tami Trivonovich, Sandy Urna, Susan Westmoreland, Jean-Ellen Wood, Lee Woodruff, and Rachelle Zidar. My deepest gratitude also goes out to those who wished to speak off the record.

Last, but not least, special thanks to Karen Miller at Boing Boing, Jennifer Norton at Claiborne, Wendy Merson at Liz Claiborne, Jane Connelly Loeb at Eddie Bauer, Yvonne Haffkoss and Charles Ryan at JCPenney, and Michele Casper at Lands' End for providing many of the clothes and accessories photographed in the book; Marc Perlson at Art-Max Fabrics in New York City for supplying the fabric swatches; John Chominsky and John Kohn at Pro-Lab, Inc., New York City, for the extra effort they put into producing the black-and-white prints; legal eagle Nina Graybill; and the folks at Macmillan—Carol Hupping, Bob Shuman, Jessica Faust, and Donna Wright—for helping to ease the stress of the first-book experience.

Part 1
Dress to Impress

"I'm getting ready for work." These are hardly fighting words, and yet, if you're reading this book, you already have some sense of the importance of how you dress as you battle your way up the ladder of success. Probably the most obvious element of a person's appearance, clothing is an important and often overlooked tool that the savvy use to get ahead. Pity the poor soul who has to find out the hard way what those who do the hiring and firing already know: that jobs have been won when the right suit was worn, promotions lost when it wasn't.

Complicating matters is the fact that office dress is going through a dramatic transition. Much of today's workforce is dressing more casually than in years past. But as you may have noticed, the rules haven't changed for everyone in every job; even within the same company, not every employee is expected to follow the same dress code.

It's for everyone who wants to dress appropriately on the job that this section was written. In the Chapter 1, "Clothes Make the Man (and Woman)," you'll discover the dramatic impact your appearance has on the impression you create—and learn how to ensure that the image you project is a winning one. Next, in Chapter 2, "The Unbuttoning of American Business," you'll be briefed on the trend toward dressing down—and receive instructions on how to carry it off without losing any clout. Finally, in Chapter 3, "Dressing Like a Team Player," you'll acquire the information you need to break one of the hardest, and most important codes of all—your company's dress code.

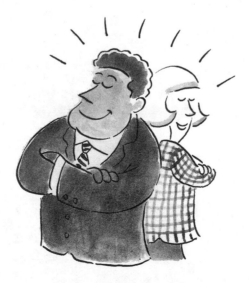

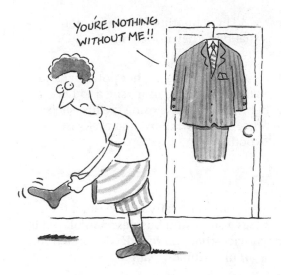

YOU'RE NOTHING WITHOUT ME!!

Chapter 1

Clothes Make the Man (and Woman)

In This Chapter

➤ Might how you look be holding you back?

➤ Packaging yourself for success

➤ Investing in your future

➤ Dressing up, moving up

➤ Must conformity cramp your style?

➤ Maintaining professionalism at home

"The apparel oft proclaims the man." —Shakespeare

Do you remember the movie *Working Girl*? It starred Melanie Griffith as Tess McGill, a bright, ambitious, hardworking woman on Wall Street who just couldn't get out of the secretarial pool. There were lots of things holding her back: She had few connections, sexist superiors, and no MBA. But her most noticeable liability was the way she looked. Her skirts were too short, her tops too tight, her hair too big. Even her patterned hosiery was too much for the ultraconservative finance industry. In short, she simply didn't look like management material.

Enter a perfectly attired, immaculately groomed new boss (Sigourney Weaver), who immediately lays down some sartorial ground rules: "I consider us a team and as such, we have a uniform—simple, elegant, impeccable." Then, quoting French fashion designer Coco Chanel, she pronounces, "Dress shabbily, they notice the dress. Dress impeccably, they notice the woman."

Taking this advice to heart, Tess sheds the downscale duds belying her potential and makes herself over into a stylish-but-serious-looking executive. Soon, she and her abilities are getting looked at in a whole new light, and by the closing credits, she's landed herself a position in management, an office with a window, and an assistant to boot. Another happy ending courtesy of Hollywood.

Dressing for Success

As much as we might like to think otherwise, this story is no fairy tale. Despite the Cinderella elements (on her way up, she also snags a successful businessman played by Harrison Ford), the underlying premise of the movie—that you're judged as much for the tailoring of your clothing as your talent—is an unfortunate reality.

The good news is that it's hardly an insurmountable obstacle. Like changing the slipcovers on a couch or repainting a room, making alterations to your appearance needn't be a full-time job or necessarily an expensive endeavor—we're not talking about cosmetic surgery here. Once you know what you're doing (something you'll learn by reading this book), it might even be fun. In any event, the payoff is too big to ignore: With the right tools (and as hard as it may be to think of suits, ties, and shoes that way, it's an accurate description), you too may find your career flourishing—or at least being recharted on a steady, upward course.

The Fashion Police

The firing line: Dress and grooming may rarely be a major factor when workers are terminated, but in a survey, one in five employers said that both had at least some impact on firing decisions.

We're So Impressionable

Consider this scary statistic: It takes less than 10 seconds to form an impression of someone. That's just slightly less time than it takes most of us to tie one shoe. Even worse than the speed with which we form impressions is the time it takes to change them. You know the old saying, A first impression is a lasting impression.

Seeing Is Believing

According to those who study this kind of thing, more than half of the initial assessment we make of someone is based on appearance—a person's age, the length of her hair, and how he's dressed. All this information is gathered and processed, before a word is ever uttered.

Now clearly, this is a flawed system. Judging someone based on a few visual clues can be dangerous. It flies in the face of all the best advice—particularly the old adage, "Don't judge a book by its cover." And yet it happens all the time! A VP who looks young for her age gets mistaken for the department secretary. A casually clad sales rep is thought to be a messenger. Oh, the indignity of it all!

What Else Is There to Go on?

Yet sometimes, especially when you're first starting out in the work world, those in the position to hire you have little else to go on than a résumé and how you present yourself. Or, in their haste to squeeze in a quick lunch between applicant interviews, they simply may not take the time to see that you're not just some average Joe or Jane—that you might be the next Bill Gates or Mrs. Fields. Only you'll know how talented you are, and you need to give potential employers and their hiring agents reason to take notice. And make no mistake: Clothes speak volumes.

Quote . . . Unquote

Clothes don't make the man, but good clothes have got many a man a good job. ...H.H. Vreeland

Of course, looking spiffy doesn't ensure your skills as an accountant or account executive—just because you can put yourself together with ease doesn't mean you can write a good sales pitch. But all things being equal, it can certainly help you get your foot in the door. A professional presentation can set you apart from the competition, and when it comes to forming impressions, it signals that you're on a fast track in the jumpstart-your-career department. Indeed, a professional appearance shows that you recognize something very important—that the exterior tells someone a lot about what's inside.

Packaging the Product—Yourself!

You don't have to have taken Marketing 101 to know that packaging can go a long way toward swaying someone to buy something. (Who hasn't bought a bottle of perfume or wine because he or she liked the label?) Of this fact, advertising agencies the world over are keenly aware. It's why boxes of detergent are blue or red (or blue and red) and not gray. It's why labels shout "new and improved" and not "same old, same old." These tactics sell!

Flex Your Marketing Muscle

Applying the principles of product packaging to how you dress and groom yourself should help you market yourself to an employer, and—provided you work hard and stay on the boss's good side—get ahead in the company.

Unfortunately, not everyone pays enough attention to his or her own sales campaign. According to a 1994 survey of readers of *Glamour*, 79 percent of women cared a lot about what to wear on a date, but only 52 percent cared as much about what they wore to work.

This admission doesn't surprise one director of human resources, who says that, sartorially speaking, most people, male and female, get too comfortable in their work environment—and she's not referring to dressing for casual Fridays. "It takes some thought to figure out what you're going to wear every day. Most people pull out all the stops for a few weeks after starting a new job, but after that, they just aim for presentable."

A Personal Appraisal

Looking professional requires that you set your standards higher, no matter what your title or profession—whether you're responsible for sharpening the boss's pencils or signing the payroll checks. Even when the economy is strong and unemployment rates are low, there's a lot of competition for the best jobs. You don't want to be held back or downsized because you look dowdy or disheveled. "Unless you have a stellar personality or wit or intellect to override how you look, not looking the part will cost you some points," notes an office manager.

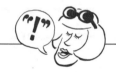

Quote . . . Unquote

How do I look from a customer point of view?...The question posed on a mirror that employees of one JCPenney store must pass several times a day.

Take a moment and assess your own packaging. What image are you projecting? Could those scuffed shoes be telegraphing a lack of attention to detail? Is that '80s power suit a sign that you're so behind the times you couldn't possibly find your own way, much less lead a staff, into the twenty-first century? Have you gotten stuck in that college groove, with hair that says, "grunge lives" or "my roommate cuts it," rather than "the perfect accouterment for my professional attire"?

Pride and Prejudice

One message your outward appearance transmits loudly and clearly is how well you think of yourself. With rare exception, a well-dressed person projects poise and conveys confidence—a winning combination in the work world. The reverse is also true. "An unprofessional appearance speaks to me of low self-esteem," says one department head. "Why would you want to do business with someone who lacks confidence?"

As teachers are known for reminding their pupils, you have to take pride in your appearance. As working stiffs, that means freshly pressed shirts and unscuffed shoes, as well as no frayed cuffs, missing buttons, chipped nail polish, or stained ties. "Pride is an important character trait, and the way a person dresses is a commentary on his or her personal pride," notes the president of an insurance brokerage.

Beyond what it says about your character, dressing well shows that you have a healthy respect for your employer and those with whom you do business. You are, after all, the company's ambassador to the outside world, so how you're perceived says a thing or two about it. As one marketing associate observes, "The first thing a client sees is you and your business card."

The Fashion Police

Big Blue's fashion coup: In the late 1930s, when salesmen were generally held in low regard, the chairman of IBM directed the sales force to wear dark suits and white shirts in an attempt to bolster their self-respect and raise their standard in the community. Did it work? You bet; just look at what an industry giant IBM became!

The Credibility Factor

Would you trust someone with a bad haircut to cut your hair? Probably not. By the same token, you wouldn't want to do business with people—whether it's buying a car from them or hiring them to do your taxes—who don't look like they can get the job done right.

One couple was put off by the sloppy showing of their mortgage broker, whom they had previously only spoken to on the phone. "His clothes were two sizes too small, his shoes were run down, his hair was hanging in his face, and here he was trying to secure a loan for us. He didn't look at all the way we expected someone who conducts major financial transactions to look. Frankly, we were relieved that he was dealing with the bank officer over the phone!"

That the broker ultimately made a costly error annoyed but didn't really surprise them; his appearance had shaken their faith in his ability, and ultimately, they steered others away from him and his firm.

Of course, not everyone who's inattentive to his or her appearance is incompetent or unreliable. But, given the option, people prefer to work with those who present themselves in a professional manner. Such has been the experience of one realtor, who credits her success as one of her firm's top producers in large part to the tailored style of dress she's adapted. "I work with people who are making the biggest investment of their life. If I don't look a certain way when explaining why a particular house is a good choice, I lose my credibility."

The Fashion Police

In the 1956 movie *The Man in the Gray Flannel Suit,* Gregory Peck's character tells a friend that he wouldn't be interested in a job in public relations because he doesn't know much about the field. "Who does?" asks the friend. "You got a clean shirt. You bathe every day. That's all there is to it." If only it were so easy!

Style Over Substance

As difficult as it is to ignore the fact that dressing successfully pays off—"It has one of the greatest returns on investment of anything you purchase," posits one professional—there may be at least a small part of you that wonders what all the fuss is about. I'm smart, you say. I'm a hard worker. Isn't that enough? Isn't all this subterfuge just a bit dishonest?

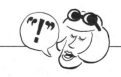

Quote . . . Unquote

Clothes make the man. Naked people have little or no influence in society. ...Mark Twain

In a word, no. Though Thoreau said to distrust any enterprise that requires new clothes, few of us live or work on Walden Pond. (And, for the record, Thoreau held only one steady job in his whole life—running his father's pencil factory for a year.) We earn our living in the real world, where people are judged not only for the quality of their work and ideas but also by what they wear. Spiffing up your personal packaging to gain a professional edge is simply a good strategic move, a close cousin to arranging your résumé so that an obvious gap between jobs seems less so. Think of it as survival of the fittest. And don't worry: Deep down inside, you'll still be you; you'll just have a nicer exterior!

Not Necessarily an Expensive Proposition

If all this talk of successful dressing is making you see dollar signs, be assured: Dressing well doesn't necessarily mean breaking the bank. Lots of successfully completed projects had small budgets—they simply required more imagination and a well-thought-out business plan. Even if you're starting from scratch, with a small but versatile wardrobe (which this book will help you choose), you can look like a million bucks by spending just a fraction of that amount!

No one has pulled off this feat better than my friend Hank. Now the owner of a small advertising firm, there was a time when his wardrobe dollar was stretched pretty thin. But from the start, he told himself that he was going to look great in whatever he wore. His secret, besides shopping the sales? "I paid attention to details. Even when I wore very inexpensive clothes, I found the best quality for my dollar and was sure that they fit just so." His other hallmark: cuff links, an accessory that instantly increases the perceived cost and elegance quotient of an outfit.

Of course, Hank's biggest professional asset is his self-assurance, the I-can-handle-anything-you-can-throw-at-me quality that he radiates. Turns out this trait isn't necessarily something a person is born with; it can be a side benefit to dressing well—like getting a gift with purchase. Says Henry, "Even if you have butterflies in your stomach, being dressing well will make you appear more confident and more in command of a situation."

Fashion Footnote

Confidence is the trait of a successful image that men most desire, according to psychologist Ross E. Goldstein, Ph.D., who surveyed more than 500 American men for Levi Strauss.

Quote . . . Unquote

Nothing succeeds like the appearance of success. ...Christopher Lascl

How Much Should You Spend?

Obviously, the more you have, the more you can spend. But in general, financial advisors suggest that no more than 5 percent of your annual income be earmarked for work clothes. So if you're earning $15,000 a year, you should allocate around $750 for your wardrobe.

Of course if you already have a job and a steady income, it's easier to budget in some new clothes. Building a wardrobe is more difficult when you're unemployed, have college loans (or Billy's orthodontia bills) to pay, or are starting from scratch. The obvious solution is to say, "Charge it." Now, I'm not suggesting that anyone go into serious debt to buy career clothing; you certainly don't want collection agencies coming after you! On the other hand, shortchanging your professional image is rather shortsighted—you need to invest in your work clothes just as you invested in your education. The best solution is to determine a budget that's realistic in terms of your own financial situation but takes into account the potential return on investment.

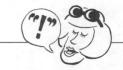

Quote . . . Unquote

You'd be surprised how much it costs to look this cheap. ...Dolly Parton

Dress for the Fast Track

Getting a promotion doesn't just mean you're able to do the work at the next level. It requires that you look the part; hence the advice to always, always, always dress as if you were in the job to which you aspire. "The daily impression you get of people tells you whether they're interested in moving up or just doing the job they were hired to do," says a human resources manager. "If you dress beyond your job when you're in a junior position, people will look at you differently."

How does that thinking square with the don't-break-the-bank philosophy of money management? Well, the idea isn't to necessarily mimic the exact look of those in the position you want, but rather to take cues from them, noting and then adopting the generalities. How long are skirts? Do men always wear jackets and ties? Do women ever wear pants? Would it be the kiss of death to wear something trendy?

Once you get the look figured out, stick with it. Having a style that fluctuates wildly won't exactly reinforce the message that you're consistent and dependable. You don't want to miss your chance to become the liaison with an important client because every other day you wear casual leggings instead of snappy separates.

Keeping You at the Top of Your Game

Whether you're consciously aware of it or not, you may also be in danger of losing your edge when you work outfit isn't up to snuff. "To tell you the truth, I do better when I think I look sharp. Even though people can't see me, *I* can see me. My energy level soars, so I come across peppier," notes a telemarketer.

It's far easier to have a winning attitude when you look like a winner, a lesson a fundraiser first learned in college. "Our soccer coach struggled mightly for several years with lousy uniforms and finally, when he had a team that was winning, he was able to persuade the college to get us new uniforms. I remember him opening up the box and saying, 'you'll perform even better when you feel good about how you're dressing.' I've never forgotten that and, as a result, I place a lot of importance on how I dress— whether I'm asking someone to donate $500,000 to improve the facilities of a pediatric intensive-care unit or just strategizing to ask for those big gifts."

Any Room for Creative Expression?

It's one of the least appealing aspects of dressing for success, the idea that you have to conform to the dictates of the company or industry in which you work. Whether you're handed a written copy of the dress code, given an verbal account or simply left to pick up on the details via your own powers of observation, there's little doubt that you're expected to follow it.

The Fashion Police

Dressing to reflect your ambition may be difficult if it involves dressing better or markedly different than your friends, family, and co-workers—a change that may upset, threaten, or mystify them. "You look classy—did you have to go to traffic court?" asked Tess McGill's fisherman boyfriend in *Working Girl,* when he saw her in sophisticated new work clothes. Not only didn't he understand the critical link between appearance and career success in corporate America he—like her best friend, a woman who took administrative style to a new low—was anything but supportive of her efforts to upgrade her image. Unfortunately, these scenarios aren't uncommon—so be forewarned!

That doesn't mean, however, that you can't express you personal style or aspects of your identity through your clothing. You're not in the Army, for Pete's sake; everyone isn't expected to look exactly alike! The key to personalizing your look is to temper your efforts so that they also reflect the particular environment in which you work. Though this is obviously easier in more creative fields, where employees are given freer range in how they dress, there's certainly room for personal expression even in typically conservative industries—though it's usually more appropriate in smaller doses, like a colorful scarf, elegant pocket square, or antique watch.

Finding a Perfect Fit

Perhaps a bigger issue is whether you can feel comfortable enough with the style of dress that your work environment demands. If not, if your preferred mode of dressing is too much at odds with what is expected of you, it could be a sign of trouble. For instance, if you're the dressy type that prefers tailored suits and crisp, cotton shirts, an organization where polo shirts and khakis are worn every day might not be right for you.

Such was the situation recently reported by the *New York Times* of a man who had left corporate America and was considering joining a small, start-up company. He had reservations, including the fact that while he was wearing a $1,000 suit at a meeting, everyone else was in shorts and sandals. (That this fledging operation had filthy restrooms and no receptionist didn't help.) Wisely, he decided to narrow his focus to more "established" companies.

Even more common is the reverse situation, where employees are annoyed about having to dress in a manner that they don't find necessary to complete their work. "The idea that I have to wear a suit or dress with pantyhose to sit behind a desk all day bugs me," notes one account executive. Ditto an accountant who has to wear a tie. "I work just as hard without one, and I'm more comfortable."

Better than realizing two months into a job at a conservative company how much you use your clothes as an outlet to express your creativity (or how absolutely constricted you feel in a suit and tie), consider what type of dress code best suits you *before* accepting a position. Feeling comfortable in your clothes and good about how you look is a critical component in how well you perform your job—and how happy you are while doing it. "If you really thrive on expressing your creativity through your costume, it may not be enough that your co-workers are creative and upbeat while wearing their conservative suits," notes a human resources manager.

Indeed, the more frustrated you become with the day-in, day-out grind of wearing clothes that you hate, the more likely it is that you will come to resent the rules—and those that enforce them. And no matter how much you may believe otherwise, chances are slim that the dress code is ever going to change radically enough to suit you. Though, you never know. A graphic artist recently influenced a small agency of slovenly employees with her professional style. "They wore sweatshirts and had uncombed hair, and there I was in my brand-new pantsuit all dressed for business. But I refused to bend." Since she's been there, the rest of the staff has raised its level of dressing to meet hers.

Working Women: No Longer Dressing Like the Men

In case you didn't get the memo, women no longer need to dress in the classic dress-for-success mode, in which their attire mirrored that of their male co-worker—a dark man-tailored suit, button-down shirt, and floppy bow tie. Honestly, back when I was starting out in the working world in the mid-1980s, women looked so mannish you could barely tell the two sexes apart!

That, of course, was the idea. Back then, women were struggling to find equal footing on traditional male turf, and the most expedient way, it seemed, was to remove any impediment—including being seen as a woman. For that period of time, the "uniform" served its purpose, but as women moved up the ranks and proved themselves to be competent professionals, the need for it has—thankfully—waned; in fact, sporting such an outdated outfit can create an impression all right, one that signals a lack of sophistication and confidence.

Today, as we head into the new millenium, there are many work-appropriate clothing options available to women—none of which compromise their credentials or hide their femininity. Still, because women have so many more clothing choices to weed through, dressing appropriately can be trickier for them. But not to worry, this book will help you choose the attire that sends the right message.

When Your Home Is Your Office

If you're one of the 40 million people who work from home (even part of the time), you may be thinking that all this dress-for-success stuff doesn't apply to you, that one of the perks of working at home is being able to wear your bathrobe all day long. Research, however, suggests otherwise—that taking the time to put on a get-down-to-business outfit positively affects your professionalism even when you're home alone.

The findings were the result of a study that monitored the performance of two groups of employees, both of which worked exclusively via the telephone. The members of one group adhered to a professional dress code; the other dressed as they wished, with no restrictions. At the study's end, the investigators found that members of the group wearing the relaxed clothes were less professional in conducting their over-the-phone business than the other group. They strayed from the business at hand more often and had conversations that were more personal in nature.

To overcome this tendency to lose sight of your purpose when relaxed to the max, consider dressing for "home" work—to mentally help you make the distinction between being at home and being at work. (One freelancing friend designates certain clothes for work and even goes so far as to apply some makeup and spritz herself with perfume. "It makes me feel better—even if nobody sees me but me!") Then, at the end of the work day, do what your office counterparts do—change into your off-duty clothes.

The Least You Need to Know

➤ How you dress is an important tool in getting ahead professionally.

➤ Impressions based in large part on your appearance are formed in a flash.

➤ It pays to assess and, if need be, to alter your personal packaging.

➤ Women in the workforce no longer have to dress like their male counterparts. Today, they can dress in a feminine fashion and still maintain their credibility.

➤ Dressing professionally doesn't have to cost a mint, nor does it require you to sacrifice your personal style.

➤ Even at-home workers benefit from dressing up; they're more productive and act more professional.

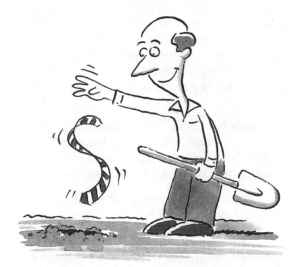

Chapter 2

The Unbuttoning of American Business

In This Chapter

➤ Casual dress: Coming soon to an office near you

➤ Casual dressing defined

➤ The do's and don'ts of dressing down

➤ Getting it right every time

As beauty director at a major woman's magazine, I was occasionally asked to make sales presentations to potential advertisers. A couple of years ago, I was slated to speak to a group of decision makers at their office on a Friday morning. For this, my first major solo effort at helping to sell our magazine, I planned my presentation—and my wardrobe—well in advance. In an effort to look authoritative yet chic, I chose a navy suit paired with black heels and a black handbag.

Meeting my co-workers in the lobby of the company's building, I was relieved to see that we were all similarly attired in our go-to-meeting outfits. Unfortunately, the other team arrived looking as if they had a softball game planned for after work, causing us to feel decidedly overdressed. Much to our dismay, we found ourselves casualties of casual Friday.

A Real Dressing Down

Casual Fridays are the biggest thing to happen to office attire since John Molloy wrote his best-selling book *Dress for Success*. But they're hardly the best thing.

Although there's no question that casual makes the 8- (or 10- or 12-) hour work day more bearable, it nonetheless makes the entire exercise of dressing more difficult for all. Gone are the good old days of pulling out two matching pieces, otherwise known as a suit, and choosing a shirt or blouse to go underneath. Though this system wasn't foolproof (admit it, we've all failed from time to time), it was certainly less tricky than trying to look professional in a polo shirt.

The fact that this trend hasn't been universally adopted doesn't make dressing down any easier. Some companies remain true to their traditional, suit-and-tie ways; others permit employees to make *every* day a casual day. Sandwiched in between are those businesses that offer just a bit of latitude, allowing only one dress-down day a week.

All this flux has created a lot of anxiety: How do I dress casually without sabotaging future success? What if my job permits jeans, but they make my buttoned-up clients jumpy? Can I project a casual-yet-in-command image?

This entire chapter is devoted to addressing (and alleviating) such concerns. It looks at this new business-fashion phenomena—and explores the ins and outs of managing it to meet your own needs.

Whatever Happened to the Gray Flannel Suit?

Just as the manner in which business is conducted has evolved over time, so has how we dress to do it. The conformity and counterculture of the '50s and '60s were replaced with the cookie-cutter clothes of the '70s: the navy pinstripe suit, white shirt, and red-print tie for men; the sensible suit with a calf-length skirt and prim bow blouse for women. A decade later, in the booming '80s, a strong-shouldered suit became the business uniform.

Fashion Footnote

Dressed down, slacking off? Savvy employees have the same work ethic no matter how they're dressed.

Fast forward to the late 1990s: In a bold break from their buttoned-up past, large and small companies across the country have given employees permission to take it easy—sartorially, that is. According to a 1997 study commissioned by Levi Strauss & Co. (which, not coincidentally, sells a lot of clothing with a casual bent), a whopping 9 out of 10 workers are allowed to dress casually to work at least occasionally.

The new work uniform runs the gamut from tailored separates at conservative firms to jeans and tees at their more informal counterparts. But make no mistake, this modern dress code still requires you to dress for success—only now you can be more comfortable while you're doing it.

America, the Casual

It's the computer engineers in Silicon Valley who are credited with the introduction of relaxed business dress. Never a buttoned-up bunch to begin with, they went even more casual as micro-chips began to rule the world and their workdays began stretching well into the night.

Fashion Footnote

Why is Friday the designated casual day at companies that permit only one? Even though Wednesdays are often talked about as being the longest workday, relaxing the dress code on Fridays give workers a little piece of the weekend, a little early.

The concept was so well received that it began to migrate east, eventually becoming a regular feature of the workweek at companies of all types and sizes across the country. That it corresponds with an increase in the number of hours employees are logging and the corporate rise of baby boomers—who enter the work environment with a wardrobe sensibility far less stuffy than that of previous generations—is no coincidence.

The trend has spread from IBM and the Ford Motor Company to the CIA and the White House, where President Clinton instituted a dress-down policy. Even the New York Stock Exchange, one of the last bastions of conservatism, is reportedly considering a change.

The Trend of the Future

Casual Fridays are just the tip of the iceberg. The one-day-a-week practice is mushrooming, frequently turning *every* day into a casual day. That same Levi Strauss study found that 55 percent of U.S. office workers (more than 40 million people) may dress casually for work Monday through Friday—an increase of 22 percent since 1995. And trend watchers don't expect a downward turn; many call casual clothes the business dress of the future. Indeed, by the year 2000, Levi Strauss predicts that half of all U.S. corporations will allow casual dress on a full-time basis. Clearly, casual is here to stay.

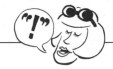

Quote . . . Unquote

Years from now, when cultural historians investigate the decline of the American empire, I am certain they will trace the collapse of a once-mighty civilization to casual Fridays. ...Joe Queenan

A Boon for Business

Even though the new code has been widely adopted, some people had concerns at first. Would relaxed clothing cause lax work habits? Would suspending a long-prescribed dress code undermine a company's establishment ethos?

17

Fashion Footnote

Hey, big spender! According to retailers, of the two genders, men are the bigger buyers of casual clothes. First, because their closets were often filled with suits and ties or jeans and T-shirts and little in between, they must make more of an initial outlay. Second, as they begin to appreciate the creative expression casual clothing affords, men can't seem to resist stocking up.

Well, as it turns out, there have been some problems (more on those later), but all in all, going casual has been good for business. "It eliminates the 'us' and 'them' mentality that we used to see between managers and the workers on the floor," notes a shift supervisor. "Now we think of ourselves more as a team. Our employees work just as hard when dressed down," says the CEO of a financial services provider, "but they appear to be happier—something that's reflected in their day-to-day contact with clients."

This sentiment is widely shared. Of the 30,000 human resource managers who participated in the Levi Strauss study, 85 percent believe that dressing casually at work improves employee morale, half say it improves productivity, and two-thirds believe it can be used as an incentive to attract new employees.

Employee-Friendly Fashion

They're not laboring under any false impressions. Surveys conducted by the *Daily News Record*, a fashion trade publication, show that employees prefer the new dress code. "This may sound extreme—it's not as though a suit is as restrictive as a straightjacket. But not being constrained by one allows my thoughts to flow more freely," says an architect, who also appreciates the ease with which more casual duds travel from the office to the work site. For one receptionist, it's almost as good as receiving a raise. "I think of it as an extra perk, like getting a few more days of vacation."

Dress-Down Daze

If the good news is that casual dress codes foster more creativity, the bad news is that less structure can create a dressing dilemma. How do people who own just two kinds of clothes—those they wear to work and those they wear at home—find a work-worthy middle ground? What exactly, they wonder, is considered appropriate? And even more important, will wearing denim do them in professionally?

The Fashion Police

Because women are still struggling to attain equality in the workplace, they should be that much more conscious of the authority-diminishing potential of dressing casually.

Employees have good reason to ponder this new policy. It requires a certain fashion finesse. Go too far, and you may see your professional image plummet. One anxious purchasing agent skirts the issue by scheduling meetings on casual Fridays so that she can wear a suit. "The excuse I give is that I don't want our vendors to feel uncomfortable. So far, my ploy is working."

A better strategy is to find out what kind of apparel works at your company on casual days. Unfortunately, a lot of businesses haven't furnished employees with a dress code for dressing down. And even when they do provide such a blueprint, it's often filled with references to "appropriate attire" but fails to adequately define it. For instance, this statement from a university in the Southeast describes only what *not* to wear:

Dollars & Sense

Employees reap some significant financial rewards while being at ease on the job. For starters, denim shirts and khakis—the outfit that's been widely adopted as the business casual uniform—cost less than suits and dresses, and they moonlight as après-office attire. Moreover, because casual clothing is oftentimes machine washable, there's usually a drop in dry-cleaning bills.

> *Regardless of the weather, it's good to remember what is considered appropriate casual dress for work on Casual Dress Fridays. Appropriate casual dress is attire that is suitable to conduct University business and to interact with the public as an employee representing the University. Appropriate casual dress specifically excludes short shorts, bare feet, halter tops, torn jeans, torn tee shirts, and the like.*

A Recipe for Success

When dressing for casual days, your goal should be to wear what makes you feel the most comfortable without compromising your credibility. Hence, casual should never be mistaken for careless. When you're just testing the waters, don't risk too much experimentation; now is not the time to show just how creative you can be. Some good rules of thumb:

1. Get your company's policy in writing—or straight from the boss. This is definitely a time when you want to hit, not miss. Besides not wanting to get a dressing down when you go too far, some companies have been known to rescind casual-day policies when employees get too relaxed.

   San Francisco Mayor Willie Brown, for instance, had employees in his office sent home, and docked pay, for coming into work in blue jeans, cutoffs or tennis shoes. (He wouldn't even speak to a tieless reporter about the matter, noting that the man "wasn't dressed properly.") On the East Coast, the Mayor of Newark, New Jersey nixed casual days when personnel showed up in halter tops and cutoff shorts.

The Fashion Police

Depending on where you work and what you do, the definition of business casual can vary widely. An iconoclastic, creative company will have fewer restrictions than traditional or conservative industries that often emphasize a particular image. Stroll around the campuses of Nike or Nintendo, and most of the workers look more like students than they do management personnel. (Other "casual" industries include journalism, filmmaking, advertising, and publishing—especially if you're on the "creative" side.) Yet visit a law, banking, accounting, or brokerage firm, and the look is decidedly less laid-back.

2. Don't equate casual with sloppy. Clothes should be clean, pressed, and well coordinated. "Too many people come to work looking like they just crawled out of bed," notes an office manager. That's because dressing down can sometimes de-motivate you. "Wearing jeans to work everyday got depressing. I started realizing that I wasn't wearing makeup or washing my hair everyday," says a woman who worked in retail display. She turned things around by buying coordinating jeans and sweaters that were casual, yet colorful.

3. Ape your boss. If you look like you're ready to hit the links and he's wearing a tweed sports jacket and nice slacks, you're underdressed.

4. Don't dress in a vacuum. Take your day's schedule—and those you're scheduled to see—into account. If you know that your company's biggest client is touring the plant or you have an appointment with a banker, you'll want to suit up—or at least take it up a notch or two. "You can't sacrifice your image by dressing casually. If I expect to represent an organization in the best light, I can't show up and say, 'Hi, I'm with this organization, and this is a worthwhile cause, but this is my casual day.' Being in my best clothes sends a message," notes a fundraiser. This thinking applies to all industries. "I'll never wear jeans on Friday if someone is coming in for an interview," notes a recruiter, whose office has a casual Friday policy. "If someone is coming to me to help them find employment, they have to trust my level of professionalism. It's a two-way street."

5. Be true to your own style. If you never wear jeans, doing so just to fit in at the office will make you feel uncomfortable.

6. What you wear on a casual workday should not be that far afield from what you wear every other day. Think of it as a more relaxed version of your Monday-through-Thursday look. So, if suits are the norm every other day of the workweek, a blazer and dressy pants might be more appropriate than jeans and a polo shirt on dress-down Fridays.

Fashion Footnote

No one dresses casually all the time. Even Bill Gates wore a suit when he testified before Congress.

7. Combine some of your existing business wardrobe with casual attire. For example, swap a sweater set for a blazer or a polo shirt for a button-down.

8. Don't assume anything. Even if you don't equate wearing pantyhose with dressing casually, your boss may.

9. When in doubt, go the conservative route. "It's always best to err on the over-dressed side. You can always remove your jacket," notes a systems analyst.

The Fashion Police

Not comfortable wearing casual? Some employees prefer dressing up. "I find that I approach my business more effectively when I really dress the part," says a bookkeeper. "Otherwise I'm more lackadaisical." Ditto an accountant who finds that dressing up helps him maintain his focus. Rather than dressing completely against the grain—you may look like you're staging a boycott—try making one small change. For a start, try scrapping the tie, trading in your leather wingtips for suede loafers, or substituting a turtlenecked sweater for a starched button-down shirt.

Anything Doesn't Go

Although every workplace environment has distinct differences in the dress code, there are similarities about what crosses the line from casual into sloppy. In general, anything you'd wear to the gym, beach, or to clean out the basement gets a thumbs-down. If you're shaking your head, thinking, geez, everyone knows that, be assured that everyone doesn't. "Sometimes employees come in wearing outfits I wouldn't even wear to McDonalds!" complains one office manager.

Business-Casual Blunders

Unless you work in an *extremely* casual environment, these will likely be considered casual-day crimes:

➤ Trendy or outrageous fashions

➤ Short or cutoff shorts

➤ Clothing with rips or holes

➤ Sweatpants and sweatshirts

➤ Baggy or very loose-fitting clothing

➤ Too tight-fitting (read: overtly sexy) clothing

➤ Tank tops, muscle tees, crop or halter tops

➤ T-shirts with slogans, pictures, or graphics

➤ Baseball caps or hats

➤ Worn-out or heavily scuffed shoes

➤ Dirty, unwashed hair

The Fashion Police

Leggings, even when worn with a blazer, are too casual for the office. "A client once spotted my co-worker in leggings and commented that, 'for a minute there I thought I had come to an exercise class.' That really hurt," reports one VP.

Quick-Change Artist

Even if you're in compliance with your office's casual-day policy, be forewarned that some situations always warrant more traditional business attire—which means you must be able to upgrade your outfit faster than you can hit the redial button on your phone. Toward this end, one company chairman reportedly changes his clothes two to three times daily to accommodate the different dress styles of those he meets.

Consider these scenarios: You've come to work wearing a T-shirt and khakis, and are asked—on the spur of the moment—to join your boss and Mr. Potential Client for lunch. Or your colleague is suddenly too tied up to make a presentation to the new recruits and asks you to pinch-hit.

What saves the day, and a lot of embarrassment for you, is the jacket, dress shirt or blouse—and if you're a guy, tie—that you keep stashed behind your office door for just such emergencies.

Paging Emily Post

A drawback to casual-day dress, as you read at the beginning of this chapter, is that there are still a lot of holdouts. The upshot: Whether you have appointments outside the office or are seeing people on your turf, your dress styles won't always be in synch—a situation that could turn awkward or embarrassing. To avoid such dress distress, a few words about casual-day etiquette are in order.

Call for the Code

When you're the one venturing into unknown territory, you may want to call ahead to the company you'll be visiting, ask what the dress code is, and then plan accordingly. (These what-are-you-going-to-be-wearing calls are fast becoming standard operating procedure.) If there's no way to get this information without losing face, send out an SOS to a friend or colleague in the know.

Give a Heads-Up

To avoid making visitors uneasy, it's helpful to alert them to your dress policy. To get the message across, one publishing firm posts signs around the office every Friday that read, "Our employees are enjoying casual day today." Many companies wisely take this one step further by requiring that their employees warn guests in advance of its dress-down days. "It's a courtesy," says an administrative assistant at a pharmaceutical company. "That way, no one feels awkward."

The Least You Need to Know

➤ The trend toward casual dress is growing; by the end of the century, it's estimated that half of U.S. corporations will permit employees to dress down every working day.

➤ What passes for casual depends on a company's culture.

➤ Think of your casual-day clothes as a relaxed version of your business style.

➤ Plan how you'll dress for work based on what you're doing that day. If you're meeting with a stuffy customer who's always suited up, dress accordingly.

➤ Providing advance warning of your company's dress code prevents visitors from feeling under- or overdressed.

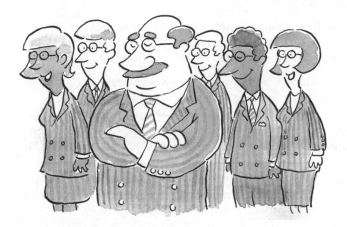

Dressing Like a Team Player

The ability to conform is not generally considered a trait of the successful. However, when it comes to dressing, original thinking isn't always rewarded. In fact, you can actually lose points if you outfit yourself much differently than your peers.

I learned this lesson firsthand a number of years ago, after accepting a job in Tennessee. Suddenly, I found myself living in a region of the country where the all-black wardrobe that had worked so effortlessly back in New York City didn't work at all. Recognizing that to my co-workers I probably looked as though I was in a continuous state of mourning, I began rethinking my wardrobe—adding more colorful clothes and limiting myself to one black piece at a time.

Though it wasn't a calculated career move, my effort didn't go unnoticed. After a few days of sporting separates in less-solemn shades, my boss commented on the change, noting that my willingness to get in step with the rest of the company reflected well on my ability to adapt. What pleased me more, however, was that it also made me feel more comfortable in my new surroundings.

The Importance of Fitting in

Sticking out like a sore thumb is hardly a goal to which anyone aspires, and yet with today's crazy quilt of acceptable business dress, it's the rare person who hasn't felt like he or she was on the wrong side of appropriate at one time or another.

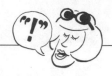

Quote . . . Unquote

When in Rome, do as the Romans do. ...allegedly Saint Ambrose said to Saint Augustine

Take Amanda, a young woman who wore a stodgy business suit to an interview at a hip ad agency. Or Mark, a financial planner who—while on vacation in Hawaii—wore his pinstriped suit to call on a client who dressed for work in flowered shirts and cotton shorts. Or Denise who, miscalculating the casual quotient of dress-down Fridays at her new job in hospital administration, came attired in an arm- and shoulder-baring tank top and blue jeans.

No matter how steely your resolve, it's impossible not to feel self-conscious in such situations. At precisely the moment you want to be sending the message, "I want to be on your team and can play by your rules," you signal that you're not even sure what game is being played!

Culture Shock

Even though Amanda's intention was to show how seriously she took the interview, in retrospect, she understands how difficult it was for the interviewer to consider her for the job. "I just didn't look like I'd fit in such an innovative environment. There wasn't anything about how I was dressed to indicate that I had a creative bone in my body."

Fashion Footnote

A winning strategy, despite the outcome: When millionaire Lamar Alexander ran for president in 1996, he began wearing lumberjack shirts as part of a strategy to connect with working-class voters.

What Amanda learned the hard way is how crucial it is that your attire mirror that of an organization's, be it formal or casual. Dressing as other employees do reflects your understanding of the company's *culture*, which is defined as the shared attitudes, values, goals, and practices of that organization—but is more simply explained as "the way things are done around here." For better or worse, how you dress is one of the easiest ways to determine if your way is the company's way. If not, says one human resource manager, it can signal rough seas ahead. "Those who don't fit in often don't succeed." The trick is identifying what's correct at your company.

Cracking the Code

Whether you're new to the workforce, relocating to another part of the country, or changing careers or companies, you may be faced with a big question: How should I dress? With business dress turned on its ear, it can be a difficult question to answer. Still, there are ways of helping you to gauge which fashions will fly at a particular organization.

What's Your Line?

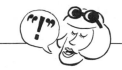

Quote . . . Unquote

Suit thyself to the estate in which thy lot is cast. ...Marcus Aurelius Antoninus

As risky as it is to stereotype, there's no doubt that some fields require conservative attire, while others demand more creative garb. For instance, in areas like entertainment, design, and fashion, there are often no limits on how imaginatively an employee dresses. "We're in the business of creativity and our clothing should reflect that," points out one graphic designer.

In other professions, no matter how original the thinking may have to be, the overriding goal of clothing is to inspire confidence: Accountants and bankers dress to convey an impression of fiscal prudence, insurance brokers to radiate reliability—so that clients feel they're in the proverbial good hands. By the same token, attorneys need to look like they can successfully maneuver their way through judicial quagmires. As a rule, all four professions require traditional attire that reflects their serious nature and historically conservative culture.

Even if you work in an arena that's fairly stuffy, your particular position may afford you some latitude. "While banking is traditionally very conservative, there's more flexibility in the marketing, advertising, and public relations departments," notes one VP.

Less Conservative Pastures

Across the board, dress codes often loosen up considerably when an employee leaves the corporate world for a position in a smaller firm—even if he or she is performing virtually the same job. Such was the experience of a woman who left Chicago and a job in corporate communications for a national realtor for a position in New York City at a small public relations firm that handled fashion and beauty accounts. "I started on a Monday wearing my Chicago clothes, a huge collection of plain polyester shells, skirts to the knee, nude hose, and low-heel pumps. It didn't take long to figure out that it was all wrong—the girl sitting next to me was wearing sundresses and sandals. By Wednesday, I had thrown away everything but the skirts, and replaced it with funkier stuff."

Also to be expected are varying expectations in dress within a single organization, as a result of the differences in job descriptions. For instance, though a school principal may wear a suit and tie, less-structured apparel is more apropos for a preschool teacher. "We play on the floor a lot and need to be able to move around easily. A blazer is too constricting," relays one teacher, who may nonetheless wear one during parent-teacher conferences.

Exceptions to the Rule

To avoid any surprises and disappointments, don't count on not being subjected to the same rules as everyone else; even if your position is one where employees are known for dressing casually, a company may expect otherwise. "I interviewed for a job in the library of a conservative corporation and was told that I'd have to wear a suit and stockings every day, year-round. I knew that jeans wouldn't be appropriate, but I never imagined that the library staff would be expected to dress quite so conservatively," relates one woman. Ditto a computer analyst at a major medical institution in the Midwest, who is expected to be in full business attire when meeting with patients and doctors, and in dressy separates on most other occasions.

Fortunately, for many workers, a rigid set of wardrobe rules isn't necessarily the norm anymore. Instead, how you dress depends in large degree on your agenda for the day and with whom you'll be crossing paths. "If I'm delivering a speech to a group of physicians or making an office call, I always wear a suit," says a woman who maintains the physician network for a managed-care company. "But when I'm in the office doing follow-up work, I dress much more casually."

The Fashion Police

Throughout history, there actually were laws governing what people could wear. These *sumptuary laws* were enacted to distinguish class, rank, or status. It's believed that the first of these laws occurred in Roman times, when the colors of togas were carefully regulated. Whereas ordinary citizens wore plain white, only the emperor could don a purple toga.

Area Codes

As the work force has become more mobile and casual (and stores with affordable work clothes like The Gap, AnnTaylor, and Eddie Bauer have sprung up across the country), the geographical differences that used to distinguish how we dressed have grown less obvious. For instance, one friend, a banker, notes that his wardrobe didn't change a whit when he moved from Manhattan to London to Charlotte, North Carolina. Still, you can see some regional similarities in how people dress for work. A few observations:

➤ In the South, women often wear clothing that's more feminine, colorful, and dressy, and, for them, accessorizing is a serious business. "It's never too much, it's more like it's just so," notes the aforementioned banker's wife, who had the same problem with black that I had.

➤ Conversely, according to one executive who recently relocated from Nashville to San Francisco, women in the city by the bay dress decidedly more casual, yet in a very sophisticated style—pant suits or elegant separates are the norm.

➤ In the Southwest and Rocky Mountains states, it's not uncommon for business-men to wear Western-style boots and string ties with their suits.

➤ With a nod toward the unpredictable weather, Northwesterners dress in a very practical style—often wearing longer coats with hoods and shoes with waffle or rubber soles. "Not a lot of suede out here," reports an investment banker.

➤ Across the board (or should I say map?), people in regions that are less populated and more rural often dress in a less fashion-forward style that's frequently casual. "Employees look tasteful and professional, but the style of clothing they wear just isn't as up to date as more metropolitan areas," says a woman whose company had its home office in El Paso, Texas.

➤ Though it varies from industry to industry, business dress seems to become less conservative and stuffy as you move westward. According to one executive who frequently crisscrosses the country on business, "Companies on the East Coast even dress more conservatively on casual days." Not that this means everyone west of the Mississippi goes without socks when "taking a meeting." Hardly. But unless you're in a traditionally conservative profession, things generally are more relaxed.

Conservatively Speaking

Some of the most conservative cities in the country are reportedly Boston, Chicago, Atlanta, and Washington, D.C. "D.C. is extremely conservative. The men put on their suit jackets to ride the elevator to another floor. If you're a woman, you'd never go without pantyhose. And you don't see a lot of people dressed trendily," notes the director of a software firm in nearby Alexandria, Virginia.

There are exceptions, of course—based on what you do for a living and your own personal style. For instance, an attorney based in D.C., who specializes in entertain-ment law, can be as freewheeling with fashion as she desires. "Luckily, my offbeat style is well accepted in this area of law." Similarily, at a small marketing firm based in Los Angeles, the president notes that one former employee's idea of acceptable attire—a sports coat, slacks, and T-shirt—didn't cut it. "It may be surprising for California, but my employees almost always wear a tie."

The More Relaxed West and South

The Pacific Northwest seems tolerant of a more laid-back mode of dressing. "We're into long, flowing skirts and little sweater tops," reports a woman who works smack-dab in the middle of downtown Portland. But here, too, that's not a look that works across the board—especially when business is conducted face to face. For a real-estate agent who works with CEOs who are relocating to Portland, a suit is a must. "That's what my clients are used to."

The weather has a big influence on how southerners dress. "I was warned that I'd never need the clothes I wore up north. Florida is so much more casual due to the heat," says a recent transplant, who conducts special promotions in a department store. "Other than the head honchos, who sometimes wear suits, people dress very casually," says an executive from Connecticut who frequently travels to Little Rock, Arkansas. "They're also more peacocky—that is, they wear brighter colors—than we do in the New York City area." Ah, one of the few constants you can count on when using geography to determine dress codes.

Fashion Police

Once you've proven yourself, and are more comfortable in you abilities, you can take a few liberties now and again. "I never went to Capitol Hill wearing pants, but my boss—who had better established herself and had more clout—would," notes a former congressional lobbyist.

Check Out the Boss

Taking your cues from the boss is a sound strategy. Not only is it the approach that the boss undoubtedly used to propel himself upward, it's the tact he or she more than likely want employees to take—in fashion lingo, it's referred to as the trickle-down effect. "As the leader of a company, I set the tone for the image clients have of it—in both the way I conduct and present myself. It's my responsibility to set the example," says one CEO.

The Fashion Police

What to do if you're a woman and your boss is a man (or vice versa)? You have two alternatives: either follow the lead of the most senior staff member of your sex or size up the boss's wardrobe—using fabric, color, and design details as clues—and then translate his style into womenswear (or hers into menswear).

Since it's the rare underling who can emulate the boss's style dollar for dollar, just take note of the generalities and try to stay in tune. If, for example, she wears dressy slacks and a sweater on casual Friday, it would be inappropriate for you to wear jeans and a T-shirt. Likewise, if he encourages a creative, but professional look, you may want to begin following the trends more closely and rethink the club ties.

Peer Review

Chances are that your peers are diligently following the leader too. So when you're new to the job, don't be afraid to look to them for guidance or to sound them out for advice.

If, however, emulating the boss means not dressing like your peers, so be it. Unless the boss is wildly out of step with the rest of the company (say, both her boss and her boss's boss dress more casually, formally, or trendily), it's wise to follow her lead even if your peers aren't. Who's to say that their goals are the same as yours? They may be happy to be departmental assistants or file clerks until they hit retirement age. You, on the other hand, want to move up. Remember this piece of get-ahead advice: Dress for the job for which you secretly yearn.

The Fashion Police

Should you outdress the boss? Only if you're sure that your superior won't be threatened by a wardrobe that's a cut above his or her own. Otherwise, and especially if you're just one promotion away from having the boss's job, you may want to avoid upstaging him or her with more expensive ensembles.

Do Research

Whenever possible, try to see firsthand how others in your chosen field dress. Some suggestions:

➤ Attend meetings or workshops of professional associations.

➤ Thumb through industry trade magazines or newsletters, which often include photographs of individual members or attendees at industry events.

➤ Go undercover. To determine how employees at a particular company dress, scope out their building, lobby, or parking lot—if you can do so without appearing suspicious! Just don't go on a Friday, the day usually set aside for casual dressing, if you want to get a true representation of the dress code.

➤ Call a company's personnel office and anonymously ask about the dress code. Instead of trying to fake it, simply say that you're new to the industry or region and that you're calling a few companies in order to get a handle on what attire is considered appropriate.

Whatever Happened to Dress Codes?

These days, it's more the exception than the rule for a company to have a dress code prescribed down to the last detail, but if it does, that code is often printed in the employee handbook.

There are several reasons most companies don't go into more depth with their dress codes—including political correctness: Even though they have the authority to set dress codes, companies don't want to come across as biased, judgmental or discriminating—especially in today's litigation-hungry environment. Also, for the sake of maintaining harmony in the ranks, companies want to avoid putting too many restrictions on employees—something many of them don't appreciate or usually feel is unnecessary. Finally, there's the inherent difficulty for a single dress code to address the roles played by all of the employees—from behind-the-scenes support staff to those who regularly interface with clients.

Consequently, dress codes are commonly written more as mission statements than as hard-and-fast rules. As an example, here's the dress code of a to-remain-anonymous mid-size computer-services corporation in the Midwest:

> *Employees are expected to maintain the highest standards of personal cleanliness, and present a neat, professional appearance at all times. Our client's satisfaction represents the most important and challenging aspect of our business. Whether or not your job responsibilities place you in direct client contact, you represent the company with your appearance as well as your actions. The properly attired individual helps to create a favorable image for the company, to the public, and to fellow employees.*

Even though this dress code is light on specifics, it's important for employees to distill its underlying message—that how they dress is a major concern to the top brass.

Memo Me on That

Occasionally, a memorandum will be circulated about varying aspects of appearance expectations. For instance, companies that allow casual Fridays only during the summer will usually review the policy via a memo distributed a few weeks before Memorial Day.

Memos are also sometimes the means through which the higher-ups deal with sartorial slipups—practices that they don't approve of and don't want to see spread from cubicle to cubicle or floor to floor. Usually these are minor infractions to the written or understood dress code; more flagrant fouls are generally addressed on the spot by, as one woman put it, some personnel policeman or policewoman.

The Fashion Police

What's the rule on pants for women? There's no one right answer for when pants are and aren't appropriate. In some conservative industries, women report that pants either aren't permissible or are only under certain circumstances. "We recently received a directive stating that women could only wear pants as part of a matching suit," relates an employee of a Fortune 100 company. And even at companies that permit trousers, women are frequently advised by their mentors to wear skirts. As one marketing assistant was informed, "They present a more polished image."

Reel Life

There's no doubt that television permeates our lives and provides endless fodder for discussions around the water cooler. But it's perfectly clear that modeling your wardrobe after television is a recipe for how *not* to succeed in business.

This is particularly true for women. When it comes to dressing for work, good female TV role models are in short supply. While male characters are at worst guilty of looking overdressed (all the patterns actually go together, there are simply too many of them), the women are usually clad in outfits that could pass for professional only in TV land: micro-minis paired with revealing camisoles or outfits that resemble leather loungewear.

Occasionally, a TV character personifies both the heart and soul of the working woman. Mary Tyler Moore, for instance, was always the picture of professionalism, wearing clothes that women could actually imagine themselves in at the office. Ditto Murphy Brown. And I daresay that Elaine on *Seinfeld* captured the dress style of the New York City publishing crowd. Even the women on *L.A. Law* seemed to be outfitted appropriately for the times.

These days, it's slim pickings—though it seems that medical and legal dramas usually come closest to hitting the mark. Taken on the whole, it probably pays to remember that most TV shows are fictionalized versions of reality. The characters on them may succeed by dressing quirkily, but the rest of us surely won't!

The Least You Need to Know

➤ To be thought of as a team player, you need to look like one.

➤ What's considered appropriate in the workplace varies widely, but there are many ways to determine what will work at your company.

➤ Just because a company doesn't have a formal dress code doesn't mean that how you dress isn't important.

➤ Using TV characters as role models for how to dress for work is risky behavior.

Part 2
The Educated Consumer

"An educated consumer is our best customer." Such is the slogan of a retail chain in the New York City area that sells upscale and designer brands of clothing at considerable savings. It's a brilliant motto, and one to which you should subscribe. Because even if your budget doesn't permit discounted designer togs, you'll still want to be a discerning shopper—to spend your fashion dollar so wisely that from the looks of things, you've already secured the corner office. Armed with the right information, you should be able to spot a suit that will give you years of good service, know when a salesperson who tells you that a jacket is supposed to fit that way is working on commission, and recognize it when a garment—expensive or otherwise—looks downright cheap.

All this and more is what you'll learn in the next three chapters, which will instruct you in the three most critical elements in a winning wardrobe—fabric, construction, and fit.

Beginning with Chapter 4, "The Material World," you'll gain a working knowledge of textiles. Next in Chapter 5, "Quality Control," you'll learn the hallmarks of good workmanship. With the information in Chapter 6, "Fit to a 'T'," you'll find out precisely how a garment is suppose to fit, so that you can ensure that your clothing looks as if it were made especially for you—whether it cost you a tidy sum or a mere pittance.

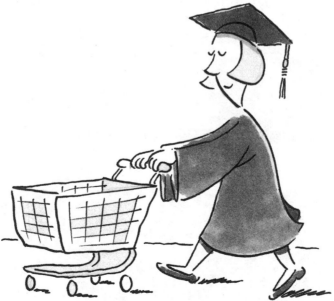

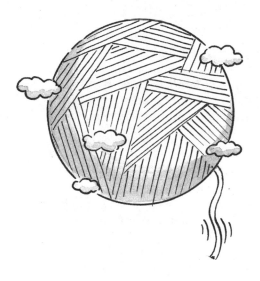

Chapter 4

The Material World

In This Chapter

➤ Fibers: natural and synthetic

➤ Fashioning fabric

➤ Hardworking fabrics

➤ The big finish

A friend in search of a new suit looked bewildered when a salesperson offered to show him a nice gabardine. Another pal ordering a polo shirt from a mail-order catalog had to ask the operator the difference between cotton piqué and jersey.

Sound familiar? Then you're in fine company. Nowadays, it's more the exception than the rule that someone can distinguish between two fabrics, and when you start tossing around terms like worsted wool and mercerized cotton, well—fuggedaboutit!

There's no doubt that textiles is a huge subject, filled with lots of lingo and technical information. Luckily, you don't need to know that much; a good understanding of the basics of fabric construction will help guide you in your selection of clothing that's fashioned of the most appropriate material—whether you're after a sport jacket that works in any climate or a blouse that needs little ironing. And that's precisely the kind of information you'll find in this chapter.

The Fiber/Fabric Connection

We tend to use the terms interchangeably, but fabrics are created when yarns of fibers—either a single type or a blend of two or more—are woven or knitted together. Any one fiber can be used to create a huge assortment of fabrics—all with different strengths, durability, weights, and textures—depending on whether and how it's woven or knitted. For example, cotton is the main component of everything from wide-wale corduroy to sturdy denim to stretchy T-shirt fabric.

There are many types of fibers: Cotton, silk, wool, and linen are natural fibers, derived from a plant or animal. Natural fibers have the irregularities and subtleties inherent in natural things, and these qualities contribute to their beauty. Rayon, acetate, nylon, and polyester are man-made, or synthetic fibers that are produced as long, spaghetti-like filaments. Until they're further treated, these fibers are smooth and slippery.

The Fashion Police

The Textile Fiber Products Identification Act requires that the fiber content of a garment and the percentage of each fiber by weight be indicated in descending order on a tag or label.

Despite these generalities, each fiber has specific properties. Knowing them will help you select garments that look, feel, and wear a certain way.

Cotton

The fibers plucked from the cotton plant have long been fashioned into some of the world's favorite fabrics—and for good reason. Though soft, cotton is extremely durable; it's the only fiber that actually becomes stronger when wet, allowing it to hold up well to repeated laundering. Cotton is also very absorbent, helping to draw moisture away from the skin. That, and the fact that it doesn't retain heat well, makes it a natural in warm and hot weather.

No fiber is perfect: Cotton's three main shortcomings are that it creases easily (though it can also withstand ironing at high temperatures) and is prone to shrinking and fading.

All cotton is not created equal. The fiber's length, which can measure from less than an inch to more than two, determines the quality of the cotton: The longer the fiber, the glossier, more resistant, and valuable it is. For instance, Egyptian and Sea Island cotton, the finest grades, average a length of 1³/₄ inches, and clothing made of it (frequently dress shirts) costs a bundle. (Pima cotton, which is also made from long-staple cotton, isn't as expensive.)

Another important distinction with cotton is whether it's combed or carded. All cotton used in clothing is *carded*, a process that removes most of the impurities and a certain amount of short or broken fibers. *Combed* cotton has undergone an extra step (thus making it more expensive) in which all the short fibers are removed. Combing produces yarn that's softer and more lustrous, even, and compact.

The Fashion Police

Cotton fabrics are frequently *preshrunk*. That is, they've been treated to inhibit shrinkage and will shrink only minimally when washed. The precise percentage of residual shrinkage is often indicated on the label. If not preshrunk, garments made of cotton can shrink as much as a full size if not properly laundered.

Linen

Yarn and fabric derived from the flax plant are known as linen. The oldest textile fiber known to man (evidence of its use dates back 10,000 years), linen can be woven into fabrics that are sheer and fine—or as coarse as canvas. Depending on the weight, linen can be cooler, stronger, and more absorbent than cotton. Poor elasticity leaves it prone to wrinkling. When combined with other fibers, linen helps improve the strength and resiliency of a finished fabric.

Silk

The handiwork of caterpillars, silk's stock-in-trade, is its brilliant luster, a trait that results from the fact that the fibers—which are secreted as fine filaments up to a mile long—are triangularly shaped and reflect light like prisms.

Despite its reputation, silk is not an especially delicate fiber; though very soft, it's actually very strong (one filament is mightier than a comparable strand of steel). It's also seasonless, keeping you cool during the summer and warm during the

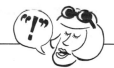

Quote . . . Unquote

Silk is the fabric you have to wear if you want to reach God. ...Ancient Chinese saying winter. Silk is naturally wrinkle-resistant; high-quality silk sheds wrinkles with a little steaming, doesn't shrink, and can go a number of wearings between cleanings because it sheds dirt.

Wool

There's a lot to love about wool. When used in high concentrations in fabrics, it meets all the qualifications for on-the-job wear. For instance:

Fashion Footnote

Pure silk is fiber to which no materials that would increase its weight have been added. It's not necessarily an indicator of better quality.

➤ It is inherently elastic, so it resists creasing and wrinkling.

➤ When it does get rumpled, the offending crimps are easily removed by pressing. (And once a new crease is set into a garment via heat, it doesn't budge until steamed out.)

➤ Though flexible, wool doesn't stretch or sag out of shape.

➤ It's easy to care for: Dirt and spills sit atop the surface of wool fabrics, where they can be brushed away or blotted.

➤ It holds up well to wear and tear.

➤ It adapts to the climate, providing warmth in the winter (the fibers trap air, creating an insulating effect) and absorbing moisture in the summer.

Perhaps the only downsides to wool are its tendencies to shrink if improperly cleaned and to form pills, those small balls of fiber that pop up on the surface—particularly in areas of friction, such as where the arms rub against the sides.

Though all wool comes from the fleece of sheep, fiber-content labels will sometimes say that a garment is made of a particular kind of wool, say, worsted or virgin. What does each term mean?

➤ **Lambswool**—Wool that comes from the first shearing of a lamb; it's very soft and has wavy fibers.

➤ **Merino wool**—A fine, high-quality wool yarn sheared from Merino sheep.

➤ **Reprocessed wool**—Wool that's been previously woven, but not worn.

➤ **Superfine wool**—The finest classification of wool, it's comparable to cashmere. Superfine wool, the finest of which is graded "Super 100," comes from strains of Merino sheep.

➤ **Virgin wool**—Wool that's being used for the first time.

Fashion Footnote

The Woolmark label identifies fabrics and/or yarns that are made from 100 percent new wool.

➤ **Worsted wool**—Wool that's made up of the harder, smoother, longer, and stronger yarns, it imparts a smooth, crisp look and feel to fabric; woolen yarns—those fashioned of shorter, twisted yarns—are more pliable, less expensive, and create fuzzier fabrics.

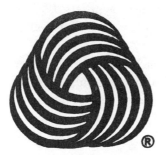

The Woolmark label indicates that fabrics have met standards for such qualities as colorfastness and resistance to pilling and abrasion. (Used with permission of The Wool Bureau.)

Rayon

Rayon straddles the divide between natural and synthetic fibers. Though composed of a material derived from trees and plants, the fibers are actually manufactured by man. Rayon, which was originally dubbed "artificial silk," shares many of the qualities of that much costlier fiber: rayon is soft, supple, lustrous, strong, and highly absorbent, and it can mimic all the other natural fibers. Viscose is the most common type of rayon.

Test-Tube Textiles

Though dyed-in-the-wool naturalists have long looked down their noses at synthetic fibers, which

Fashion Footnote

"Blended" yarns combine the most desirable features of several fibers. For instance, one very popular combination, wool/polyester blend, provides the drapability of wool and the strength and wearability of polyester.

are mostly created from chemicals, they're anything but second-class materials. Indeed, when combined with natural fibers, synthetic fibers enhance the overall performance and practicality of a fabric. How so? By making them wrinkle resistant, easier to care for, and longer lasting. Here's a rundown of technology's top offerings:

➤ **Acetate**—Like rayon, acetate is a hybrid, a synthetic fiber with natural roots. Used during World War I to make waterproof varnishes, today it's called into action when a lightweight, silky fabric is needed. Fabrics made of 100 percent acetate are often used to line garments.

➤ **Acrylic**—A strong, warm fabric that drapes well, acrylic is often used as a synthetic substitute for wool.

➤ **Microfibers**—Polyester or nylon fibers that, as their name implies, have much smaller diameters than their traditional counterparts. The beauty of microfibers is

41

the rich, soft, silklike feel they provide without sacrificing their other more utilitarian qualities. These days, everything from pantyhose to trench coats are made of microfibers.

➤ **Nylon**—A high-strength, quick-drying, elastic fiber.

➤ **Polyester**—One of the most frequently used synthetic fibers in clothing due to the fact that it keeps its shape, resists creasing, wears well, and is a breeze to care for.

➤ **Spandex**—A strong fiber that adds stretch and holding power to fabrics. (Spandex can stretch as much as 500 percent without breaking.) Even a small percentage of spandex in a garment (as little as 5 percent) will do the trick. Lycra is the trademark for spandex made by DuPont.

➤ **Triacetate**—A relative of acetate; its ability to better tolerate heat means it can be ironed at higher temperatures.

The Fashion Police

Synthetic fibers' biggest offense is that they don't "breathe," that is, pull moisture away from the body and release it back into the environment. That's because they can't absorb moisture. While they do "wick" moisture from the body, it remains on the surface of the fabric. As a result, a garment high in synthetic fibers can feel clammy on hot days and chilly on cold ones.

Precious Fibers

They're the 24-karat gold of wool fibers, prized for their fineness, softness, and warmth—and priced in the stratosphere because of their scarcity. They can be blended into fabrics or used solo—creating the ultimate in luxury! Many are fashioned into suits, sweaters, coats, and more affordable accessories like gloves and scarves.

➤ **Alpaca**—Fleece derived from the Alpaca, a member of the camel family that's bred in Peru. Fabrics made from alpaca are warm, lightweight, with a silky-soft hand, and good draping properties.

➤ **Camel hair**—The thick, soft undercoat of the Bactrian camel of Asia, collected after the animal sheds or is sheared.

➤ **Cashmere**—The fine, downy-soft undergrowth produced by the cashmere goat.

➤ **Mohair**—A long, white, lustrous hair obtained from the Angora goat. (The fabric referred to as angora actually comes from the Angora rabbit.)

➤ **Vicuña**—The finest of all animal fibers, vicuña is soft, strong, and expensive to produce—it takes a dozen vicuñas, a small animal of the llama family, to make one piece of cloth. Because vicuñas are so wild, they must be killed in order for their hair to be obtained.

The Ways of Weaving

Though there are variations on each theme, fibers are woven into fabrics via one of three basic weaves—plain, twill, and satin. Certain characteristics are common to each type.

1. The **plain weave** is the simplest, and most commonly used, accounting for 80 percent of woven fabrics. Its effect resembles a checkerboard pattern. Examples of plain fabrics: oxford cloth, chambray, seersucker, and poplin.

2. The **twill weave** is a very durable weave that's characterized by the diagonal ribs that form on one or both sides of the fabric. Examples of twill fabrics: gabardine, serge, and denim.

3. The **satin weave** produces a subtle sheen and luxurious drape. Example of satin fabrics: sateen.

Fashion Footnote

In textile talk, "hand" refers to the way a fabric feels (for instance, how soft or stiff it is), while "body" is used to describe the solid, compact feel of fabrics. "Drape" has to do with the way a fabric falls when hung or arranged in a different position. A very supple, flexible fabric is said to drape well.

The Knitting Factory

Fabrics that aren't woven are usually knitted, either by a hand knitter using two needles or by a high-speed knitting machine. Either way, the same basic technique is used to create knits: Rows of loops are interlaced using a variety of stitches. Knitted fabrics will usually "give" (which is why they're often so comfortable), though their ability to do so depends on both the type of stitch and the yarn used.

Knitspeak

Even if you don't know what *purl* means, you should be aware of the following knitting terms:

➤ **Argyle**—A multicolored, diamond pattern knitted into socks and sweaters.

➤ **Cable knit**—A raised, decorative pattern resembling twisted cables that's frequently used in sweaters.

➤ **Interlock**—A fine-gauge fabric in which the front and back of the fabric look identical.

➤ **Jersey**—A soft, smooth, stretchable fabric without a distinct rib.

➤ **Rib knit**—Fabrics with lengthwise ribs of any width; rib knitting is heavier, and more durable and elastic (especially in the crosswise direction), than flat knitting is—making it especially suitable for cuffs and waistbands.

➤ **Tricot**—Knits that exhibit fine ribs on the front, crosswise rows on the back. They have a soft, draping quality.

Fashion Footnote

A knitted garment that's *full-fashioned* will fit better and have less-prominent seams and—as a result—be more expensive than one that's "cut-and-sewn" with the full-fashioning technique. Fabric panels are shaped during the knitting process by increasing or decreasing the number of loops; with cut-and-sew garments, panels are cut from a bolt of knit cloth and then sewn together. The hallmark of full-fashioning are "pockmarks" whenever the garment was shaped.

Why Ply?

Knitwear is often described as being anywhere from one to four ply. The term refers to the number of strands twisted to form a single yarn. The higher the number, the plusher, warmer, and thicker the garment. So, while a thin, one-ply sweater layers easily under a jacket, a sweater that's four ply works best on its own.

The Fabrics of Our Work Lives

Of the virtually thousands of fabrics known to man, a couple dozen are most commonly used to fashion our on-the-job clothing. The following guide will acquaint you with many of them.

➤ **Broadcloth**—Both a closely woven wool-suiting cloth with a smooth nap and lustrous appearance, and a tightly woven cotton or cotton-blend cloth with a fine crosswise rib that's frequently used for shirts.

➤ **Chambray**—Sort of a lightweight denim, it's also woven with colored and white threads. A popular shirting fabric, it was originally woven in Cambrai, France—hence, its name.

➤ **Challis**—A lightweight, plain woven fabric printed with a delicate floral pattern; mostly used as a dress fabric.

➤ **Corduroy**—From the French *corde du roi*, or "cloth of the king," a durable fabric with wide wales or pinwales, cords, or ribs. Although shirts, trousers, and jackets made of corduroy have a sporty look, wide-wale corduroy often looks very elegant.

➤ **Crepe**—Any fabric with a crinkly, pebbly surface. (The word crepe comes from the French term, *créu*, meaning crimped or wrinkled.) Crepes have a dressy feel, drape well, and are good at resisting wrinkles.

➤ **Denim**—If you own a pair of jeans, you own some denim. A rugged, cotton twill fabric, it comes in many colors as well as the original indigo blue. Its name is derived from Nîmes, France, the town in which it originated.

➤ **Flannel**—A softly brushed fabric, often made of worsted wool, that lends a casual, sporty look to blazers or trousers. (Don't mistake it for the cotton flannel used to make PJ's.) The downside of flannel is that it's very prone to wearing out rapidly in areas subject to friction, for instance, the inner thighs.

➤ **Gabardine**—A durable, tightly woven fabric with definite diagonal ridges that can be made in a variety of weights from natural and synthetic fibers. It's the workhorse of suiting fabrics.

➤ **Khaki**—A sturdy material, historically used for military uniforms, that's a dull yellowish-brown color. (Also a style of pant that rules on casual Fridays.)

➤ **Moleskin**—A heavy, strong cotton fabric that's brushed to suede-like softness.

➤ **Oxford**—A durable fabric woven from heavy, predominantly cotton yarns. Button-down shirts are frequently made of oxford cloth.

➤ **Piqué**—A durable, knitted cotton fabric, with a waffle, or diamond shaped pattern that's produced by weaving together two cloths, one above the other. Polo shirts are often fashioned of piqué.

➤ **Poplin**—A strong, hard-wearing fabric used mostly for high-quality shirting and summer suits, it's characterized by crosswise ribs that give it a corded effect.

➤ **Seersucker**—The quintessential summer suit fabric; a lightweight, usually cotton fabric with a crinkly striped surface.

➤ **Serge**—A suiting material characterized by a flat, diagonal rib. *Serge* and *twill* are often used synonymously.

➤ **Tencel**—Trademark for a soft, natural fiber made with trees grown on managed tree farms.

➤ **Tricotene**—A fabric with a distinct double twill line, it's used for suits and sportswear.

➤ **Tropical suiting**—Lightweight, soft, fluid, usually wool fabrics that provide year-round wear. Think of them as "wool lite."

➤ **Tweed**—A general term for rough fabrics woven from wool in a variety of effects, including checks, plaids, flecks, and solids. Because of its coarseness, tweeds are usually saved for lined jackets and trousers. Harris Tweed refers to woolen fabric handwoven on the islands of the outer Hebrides off the northern coast of Scotland—including the Island of Harris.

➤ **Velvet**—A tightly woven fabric with a short, dense pile or fuzzy finish, which produces a soft, rich texture. Velveteen has a shorter, less-luxurious pile.

➤ **Viyella**—Trade name for a soft, warm, hard-wearing fabric of 55 percent wool and 45 percent cotton.

Hardworking fabrics (from top): flannel, tweed, crepe, seersucker, pinwale corduroy, khaki, wide-wale corduroy, denim.

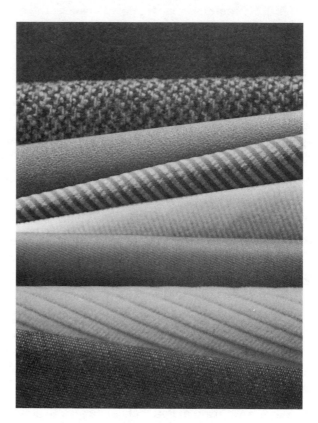

The Fashion Police

Quality fabrics feel substantial, luxurious, and nice against the skin. Lesser-grade material feels thin, scratchy, or stiff. Learn the difference by handling and comparing expensive and inexpensive materials at a fabric store.

Giving Special Treatment

Specially treating fabrics can make them more suitable for specific jobs. Some common treatments include:

➤ **Crease or wrinkle resistant**—A finish used on cotton, linen, rayon, and blended fabrics that increases resistance to and recovery from wrinkling, sometimes at the expense of comfort.

➤ **Mercerization**—Process in which cotton is treated with caustic soda. The silky, lustrous finish helps to increase the strength of the fabric.

➤ **Sanforized**—Trademark name of fabric that's been processed to prevent shrinking.

➤ **Scotchgard**—Trademark for a finish that makes fabrics resistant to grease and water stains.

➤ **Teflon**—A synthetic coating that helps fabrics repel spills and stains.

The Least You Need to Know

➤ Fibers are either woven or knitted into fabrics. Knits generally have more "give" than weaves.

➤ Natural fibers such as cotton, linen, silk, and wool are all durable, and they're comfortable to wear because they "breathe."

➤ Acetate, microfiber, spandex, and other manufactured fibers are often blended with natural fiber to make them less prone to wrinkling and easier to care for.

➤ Fabrics can be treated with various finishes—for instance, they can be mercerized or Sanfordized—to make them more user-friendly.

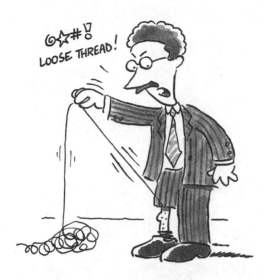

Chapter 5

Quality Control

In This Chapter

➤ Recognizing quality construction

➤ Checking out the exterior

➤ What's inside tells a lot

➤ Facts on fasteners

I always loved the slogan that Ford used to advertise its cars: "Where quality is job one." It is, no doubt, a sentiment that consumers would like to see applied to all products—and clothing is no exception. Unfortunately, quality construction in clothing is definitely not a sure thing—seams, hems, linings, and buttons often come undone after only a few washes or wears. Even paying a lot of money for a garment is no guarantee that it's well made.

So how can consumers know when they're spending wisely or overpaying for shoddy workmanship? By buying clothing that comes close to meeting a high standard of quality, you'll be assured that it's going to wear well, look good, and—most important—make you look good! Even if you're on a tight budget, you'll at least want to apply the following guidelines to those pieces for which you're forking over the most money.

At First Glance

You don't always have to look hard to see that a garment isn't up to snuff. Some details are dead giveaways. Here's a rundown.

It's a Match!

It's a sure sign of inferior quality when the plaid or other pattern on a garment doesn't match—yet you'll see it on the priciest of pieces. (*Warning:* Once you notice this, it may drive you to distraction—as it does me when watching news anchors and talking heads!). While it may cost more for them to do so (for one thing, the venture requires more fabric), patterns should align without interruption at pockets and seams. If you can't find or afford garments with matched patterns, stick with solids.

An obvious pattern should match at the shoulder, the collar, and continue across the front to the sleeve. (Pinstripe jacket courtesy of JCPenney.)

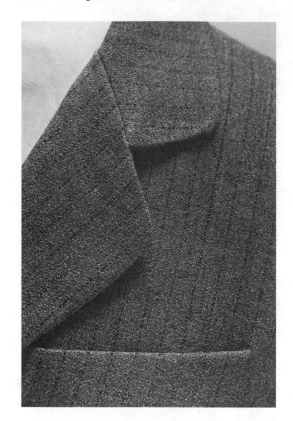

Top Collars

Whether yours are white or blue, shirt collars should lie flat, have points of equal length, and be pucker free. If the shirt fabric is patterned, the pattern on your collar should look symmetrical—meaning it should "balance," or mirror itself on the left and the right sides.

Lapel Lesson

Lapels are the vertical folds of the front of a jacket or coat that extend down from the collar. Whichever style you choose (peaked, notched, and shawl are the most common), the two sides should be symmetrical and lie flat.

Pocket Picking

The cheapest variety of pocket is the mock, stitched on kind; the presence of these fake pockets is often a tip-off that a jacket is poorly constructed.

Truly functional pockets, especially those on pants, should be deep and roomy, and ideally lined in cotton. Regardless of the type, all pockets should lie closed and never create gaps or pulls. Patch pockets, those that appear on the outside of a garment, should be reinforced with stitching at the top corners (it sometimes takes the form of a small triangle).

By the way, many pockets are stitched closed when you purchase a garment to keep them lying flat. Unless they're too small to serve much more than a decorative purpose (sometimes, especially on women's garment, pockets aren't large enough to hold much more than a tissue), open them carefully with a seam ripper.

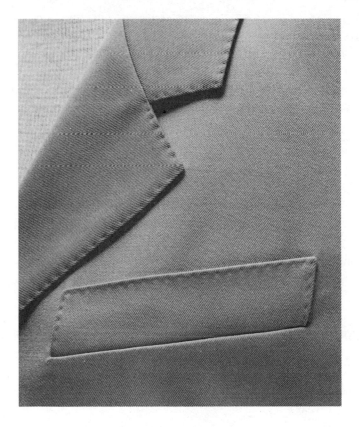

A functional handkerchief pocket is a mark of quality.

The Fashion Police

Symmetry is key to good clothing construction. Check that the length of the two front pieces of a jacket are the same by folding the jacket in half and holding the shoulder seams together.

It's Not Immaterial

No matter how well constructed a garment may be, if the fabric isn't up to snuff, you may be buying a lemon. To recognize quality material, or its opposite, you must be able to distinguish the characteristics that signify excellence—and those that disguise inferiority. The following are the most obvious to the inexperienced eye:

➤ The weave should be firm. Test this by scratching the surface. If the threads easily shift, the garment's seams may be inclined to slip or develop holes around the stitching.

➤ The weave should be uniform. Hold it up to the light and check for any unusually thick or thin areas. A fabric that has them may not wear evenly.

➤ The lengthwise and crosswise threads should meet at right angles, with the lengthwise threads running straight up and down the garment. If they don't, the fabric is off-grain and may not hang correctly—something that's particularly noticeable in prints.

➤ No powdery dust should appear when the fabric is rubbed between the fingers. Visible powder is an indication of too much sizing, a frequent device for concealing poor quality.

➤ Fabric should shed wrinkles after being squeezed for about 10 seconds, either immediately or within a few minutes. If it doesn't, the garment will always look rumpled.

➤ The fabric shouldn't easily pill, that is, produce small balls of fibers on the surface. To test, gently rub two layers of fabric right sides together. If pills form, the fabric certainly won't wear well.

The Inside Story

My high school sewing teacher always told the class that our garments should look as good on the inside as they do on the outside. No, her standards weren't ridiculously high; the thinking behind this logic is that the better a garment is made on the inside, the better it will wear. Read on for information on what to look for when you take a peek inside.

Silver Linings

In addition to concealing the inner construction of the garment by providing a neat, clean finish, a lining serves many purposes. For starters, because it acts as a buffer between the fabric and your body (smoothing over bumps and bulges), it helps a garment fit better. It also reduces wear from the inside out. And because linings are—or at least should be—made from smooth, shiny materials, they make it easier to put the garment on and take it off. There are three main considerations when evaluating a lining:

1. A lining should follow the drape of the garment and be loosely cut to allow for body movement.

2. A lining should hang smooth and not dangle below the hem.

3. A lining should be securely anchored, but not sewn at any point other than the edges—so movement isn't compromised.

In suits, the lining of the skirt and jacket should be made from the same fabric or in a color that coordinates well with the garment fabric.

Linings on women's pants are generally full length, while men's normally reach the knees. Better-quality men's trousers, whether lined or not, have an extra piece of fabric inside, from the crotch down, designed to absorb friction and extend the life of the pants.

Looking Over the Shoulder

Shoulder pads should be symmetrical: equally positioned and sized. They should also be invisible throughout the fabric. Beware any rippling at the junction where the shoulder and sleeve meet; the seam should be seamlessly stitched. If they don't sit smoothly now, they never will.

Fashion Footnote

What's a *bemberg lining?* Bemberg refers to the silky soft fabric, a type of rayon known as cuprammonium, from which top-of-the-line linings are fashioned. It's named for the German man who created it. Bemberg linings are most often found in fine men's clothing, though some women's clothing now features them.

Dollars & Sense

A jacket that's unlined isn't necessarily inferior to one with a lining. In fact, an unlined jacket may actually be more expensive, since the cost of lining pales next to the work involved in properly finishing an unlined jacket—so that it looks as good on the inside as the outside.

The shoulder area should be free of puckers.

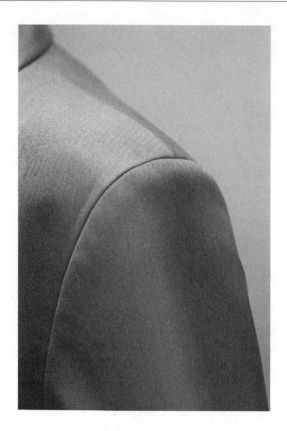

Superior Sleeves

Deep armholes makes it easier to raise and move your arms, but when they're cut too deeply—so as to accommodate a wide variety of chest and back sizes—they look awkward. A good rule of thumb is to look for an armseye that doesn't fall more than $1\frac{1}{2}$ inches below your armpit—unless the design of the garment calls for it to.

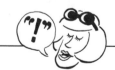

Quote . . . Unquote

Just as the chassis of a car must support the body, so the strong yet supple framework of a jacket helps it to keep its shape when worn.
...Messieurs, Summer, 1949

The Facts on Fusing

Much ado is made about whether a jacket is fused or unfused. What's the difference? Between the fabric and the lining of a jacket is a layer of reinforcement; in top-of-the-line garments, it's made of canvas and is inserted by hand, allowing for greater flexibility. The alternative—and much less expensive—method is fusing, in which a synthetic fabric with an adhesive back is attached to the inside of the outer fabric by heat. (A jacket is fused if the interfacing can't be felt as a separate layer if you pull the two layers of the lapel apart.)

In its early incarnation, fusing imparted a very stiff appearance, but improvements in fusing reportedly now permit a softer effect. Still, it varies greatly in quality. What owners of fused jackets need to be mindful of is that the excessive heat or harsh chemicals used by some dry cleaners can cause the fusing to become unattached. This condition usually results in shrinkage, bubbling, and an overall loss of shape. (If this happens to your jacket, stop wearing it. I once worked with a woman who continually wore a seriously bubbled jacket to work.) To avoid this potential problem, check out Chapter 22, "Care and Keeping," to learn how to choose a high-quality dry cleaner.

So It Seams

Seams are designed to lie flat; if they pucker, pull, or don't hang straight, it may indicate that they were sewn using incorrect tension—something that makes them weak and prone to breaking.

Especially in unlined garments, seams should be finished to keep fabric from unraveling and to add a measure of neatness. The nicest finishes completely enclose the seams.

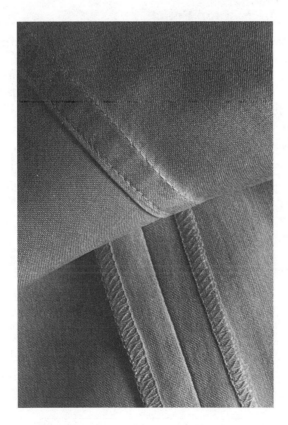

Seams should be neatly finished.

A Stitch in Time

Even in the highest-quality garments, stitching is being done less by hand (a method that provides more flexibility) and more by machine. Look for straight, even stitching that averages about 8 to 12 stitches per inch, with heavier fabrics getting longer stitches. In areas of high stress, like under the arms, it's a plus if stitches are a bit tighter.

When it comes to machine stitching, one needle is better than two. Double-needle stitching, though faster, is more likely than single-needle stitching to produce puckered seams. Shirts are often single-needle stitched, and those that are will note that fact on the packaging.

The Fashion Police

Topstitching is the stitching seen on the outside of a garment. Its presence can signal one of two things: shoddy construction, with the topstitching actually being used to help hold a garment together, or a decorative touch that signals quality and attention to detail. How do you know its purpose on a garment you're considering buying? In general, if the garment is otherwise well made, you can assume that topstitching is another hallmark of fine craftsmanship. That's certainly the case if the tiny stitching known as pickstitching is employed.

Uh-Hem!

As much as hemlines go up and down, two things about hems should remain constant: They should hang straight and even and be securely fastened and finished with tape.

The best hemline stitching is invisible or darn near close to it. If you must buy a garment with a poorly sewn or missing hem (it's not unusual for one to have been inadvertently detached while being tried on), re-hem it or have it re-hemmed using the uneven slip stitch (see Chapter 22 for how-tos).

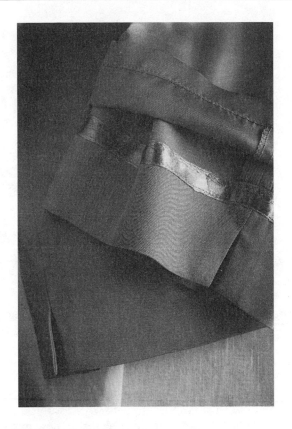

The stitching used to secure a hem shouldn't be visible to the naked eye. Hems finished with tape look neat and are especially appropriate on fabrics that ravel. (Pants courtesy of Eddie Bauer.)

Closing Arguments

Garments need to be fastened shut—for the sake of modesty, so that they stay up, or simply to keep out the cold. No matter what their purpose, some details in buttoning and zippering indicate higher quality.

Button Up

There are two basic types of buttons: sew-through and shank. The sew-through button has holes, either two or four, through which it's attached; the shank button has a solid top with a "neck" beneath to accommodate thicker fabrics and to allow the button to rest atop the buttonhole instead of crowding to the inside. In case you're wondering, when sew-through buttons have a thread-created stem between them and the fabric, it's usually a sign they've been sewn on by hand—a more secure method.

Fashion Footnote

Ladies, check to be sure that buttons are strategically placed so that a garment doesn't gape open at the bust area. The safest button position is in the center of the fullest part of the bust.

A key-shaped buttonhole makes buttoning easier. A shank between the button and the fabric creates a smoother look when a garment is closed.

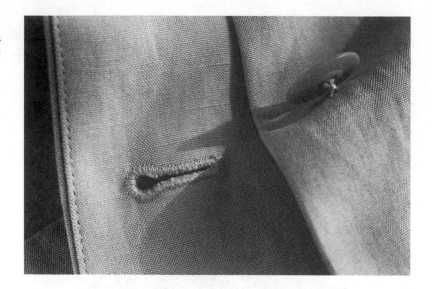

Fashion Footnote

Though their purpose is mainly decorative, buttons on the sleeve of a jacket are a nice touch—unless they're just stitched onto the fabric. At the very least, the sleeve should be vented (that is, have a vertical slit that extends three or four inches from the bottom of the sleeve), so the buttons appear to function.

The finest buttons are bone, mother-of-pearl, shell, horn, leather, polished brass, or covered; plastic buttons are cheap and will easily break and crack. Whatever material they're made of, buttons should be sewn on tightly. On thicker garments, like coats and jackets, buttons should be reinforced on the underside of the garment with small, flat buttons; by absorbing the stress that would otherwise be on the fabric, these extra buttons help keep it from tearing. If a fabric is more delicate, the underside should be reinforced with a small square of matching fabric.

The more buttons on a garment the better (some say that a man's shirt should have at least seven), and having a few spares—especially if the buttons are at all unusual and therefore, difficult to replace—is a plus. Gauntlet buttons, those situated a few inches above the cuff that keep the sleeve opening closed (and your forearm from being exposed), are a mark of quality.

When buying pants, make sure there's an extra button behind the fly area, to serve the same purpose as those small reinforcement buttons.

Finally, buttonholes should be neatly finished, either with closely spaced stitching or fabric. (On pricier garments, tight, but irregular stitching may indicate hand sewing.) Be on the lookout for loose threads, which may eventually come undone, leaving the fabric exposed and prone to fraying. The buttonhole of choice is the keyhole; its shape (an old-fashioned keyhole) makes it easier to get the button through, meaning there's less wear and tear on the fabric.

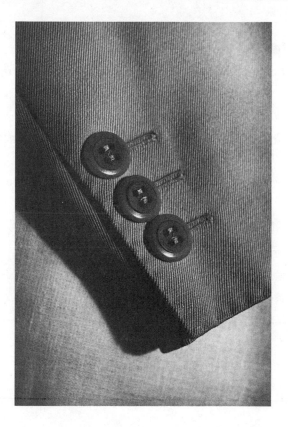

Nowadays, buttons on the sleeves are merely a nice touch, especially if they appear to work. Once upon a time, however, their purpose was to discourage soldiers from wiping their noses with their sleeves!

Zip It

Zippers should slide up and down without being impeded. If one stops and starts or needs any finessing when tested, either choose another of the same garment or be prepared to replace the faulty fastener.

Unless it somehow enhances the look of a garment, a zipper should match the predominant color of the garment and be neatly concealed.

Fashion Footnote

When you have a choice between a fly that closes with buttons or a zipper, consider the two schools of thought. Though more time-consuming to operate, purists maintain that buttons are more secure than a zipper, which can experience mechanical difficulties. On the other hand, zippers are thought to provide a more uniform effect—especially in pants made of lighter fabrics.

The Least You Need to Know

➤ A garment's construction determines not only how it will look when worn, but how well it will wear.

➤ Price is not always a good indicator of quality work.

➤ Some hallmarks of quality include even stitching, patterns that match, neatly finished seams, and symmetrical design elements.

➤ Not every piece of clothing you buy needs to be couture quality, but the ones you spend major money on should come as close as possible.

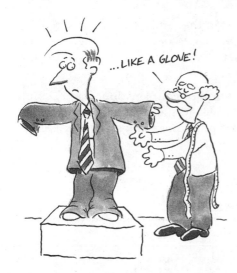

...LIKE A GLOVE!

Chapter 6

Fit to a "T"

In This Chapter

➤ Measurement-taking how-tos

➤ Sizing up sizing

➤ Fit makers and breakers

➤ Recognizing a good fit when you see it

It's one of the basic tenets of clothing: It should fit. Well. Not necessarily like a glove or even a second skin, neither of which would fly in most office environments nor be very comfortable for 10 to 12 hour stretches. But a garment should look and feel as though it was constructed for you and only you, not a taller, thinner, shorter, or stockier version of you.

If that vision doesn't exactly describe the state of your work wardrobe, it may be because you subscribe to the theory that a garment fits as long as you can get all the buttons on it closed—even if you have to suck in your stomach to do so. But alas, a well-fitted garment goes way beyond that. Indeed, to be outfitted in truly successful style, your clothing—no matter how much you paid for it—should fit just so, especially considering a poor fit can cheapen a $1,000 suit, and a good one can make a $59 jacket look custom made. What's the criteria for a good fit?

How Do You Measure Up?

The first step to getting a good fit is knowing your measurements. Though less vital for women, who have different systems of sizing, this knowledge is of tremendous importance for men, since their clothing sizes are often the same as their measurements. For instance, when a guy buys a dress shirt, it's based on two measurements—the circumference of his neck and his shirt-sleeve length. Similarly, a man's pant size comprises two measurements—his waist and inseam.

What follows is a unisex guide to obtaining a half dozen of your key dimensions. A few tips: When measuring, keep the tape comfortably loose and stand in a natural pose. Always re-measure if you gain or lose weight, or your physique changes, say, as a result of working out.

Table 6.1 Measure for Measure

Measurement	Where to Measure	
	Men	**Women**
Chest/bust	Right under the arms, around the fullest part of the chest—being sure to keep tape over the shoulder blades.	Under the arms and over the fullest part of the back and bust while wearing a bra.
Hips	Where the buttocks and legs meet, around the fullest part.	This point is usually 7 to 9 inches below your waist.
Inseam	The inside of the leg from the crotch to the desired length. Or, using a pair of pants that fit well, measure from the crotch seam to the bottom of the pant leg.	
Neck	Around the fullest part of the neck, including the Adam's apple. Add $1/2$ inch to determine your neck size.	
Shirt-sleeve length	From the neck base at the center back, along the shoulder, over the bent arm to where wrist and palm intersect.	
Waist	Around the natural waistline. If you're not sure where that is, tie a string snugly around your middle; it will roll to the natural waist.	

Sizing Up the Situation

In addition to the straightforward your-measurement-as-your-size system, there are two common approaches to sizing. One, which is used in both menswear and womenswear (though mostly for buying unstructured garments), designates two or more sizes or measurements as either small, medium, or large—or, in some cases, extra small and extra large or larger. For example, at one company, men's chest sizes 38 to 40 are designated a size medium, while women's sizes 4 to 6 are equivalent to a size small.

In the second system, which is used only in women's clothing, sizes range from 2 to 30. With this method, measurements are assigned a number—for instance, a 26-inch waist may be deemed a size 10, while a 28-inch waist is equivalent to a size 12.

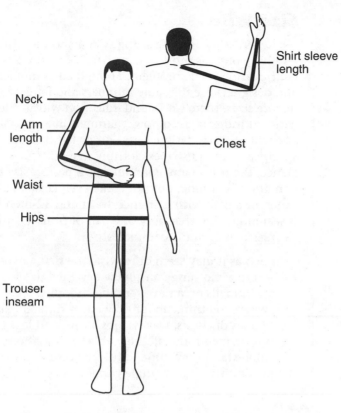

How do you measure up? Use these guides to measure your neck, chest, waist, hip, inseam, and shirt-sleeve length.

Shirt sleeve length

Neck

Arm length

Chest

Waist

Hips

Trouser inseam

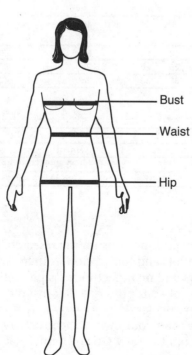

Bust

Waist

Hip

Fashion Footnote

There's more riding on how your clothing fits than just looks; your health may also be at stake. For example, too-tight trousers have been observed to be the cause of abdominal discomfort—particularly in men whose waistbands were at least 2 inches smaller than their middles. Similarly, constricting necklines—which press carotid arteries of the neck, blocking blood flow to the brain—may impair vision, according to a study conducted at Cornell University.

Size Wise

As user-friendly as these sizing systems sound, they're anything but—as most anyone who's ever bought clothes knows. The problem: Though all manufacturers and designers use the same numbers and letters to denote sizes, there's no standardization within the garment industry as to how a garment in a particular size will fit. Each designer uses his or her own set of specifications and shapes clothing in a particular way. Hence, the reason a woman may be a perfect size 8 in one line of clothing, but not come even close in another, or a man with a 38-inch waist and 32-inch inseam may find that only one pair of trousers out of four sized as such fits comfortably.

As much as it may seem otherwise, the sizing issue isn't some sort of clothing conspiracy designed to keep people in malls on a never-ending shopping spree. In fact, when you think about how many different sizes and shapes of chests, waists, hips, arms, and legs there are and then consider all the viable combinations, you can understand how difficult it is to accommodate all the possibilities in one single garment size.

Sizing varies from one clothing manufacturer to another, sometimes widely. For instance, these two size charts run anywhere from 1/2 inch smaller to an entire size larger than those from other companies. They will, however, give you a general idea of the size of you need.

Misses Sizes

Size	2	4	6	8	10	12	14	16	18
	XS	S	S	M	M	L	L	XL	XL
Bust	32	33	34	35	36	37 1/2	39	40 1/2	42 1/2
Waist	24	25	26	27	28	29 1/2	31	32 1/2	34 1/2
Hips	34	35	36	37	38	39 1/2	41	42 1/2	44 1/2

Men's Sizes

Size	S	M	L	XL
Neck	14-14 1/2	15-15 1/2	16-16 1/2	17-17 1/2
Chest	37-39	40-42	43-45	46-48
Waist	28-31	32-35	36-39	40-43

Finding the Right Size

The solution to this problem is simple, albeit time-consuming: research. It's only through trial and error (that is, trying on lots and lots of clothes in an array of sizes) that you'll discover how certain designers and manufacturers shape their clothing and how their systems match the proportions of your physique. For instance, as much as you may like the styling sensibility of a particular designer, you may find that the clothing is cut for a frame that's slimmer than your own. Or, conversely, you may end up looking like you're wearing castoffs from the Jolly Green Giant. That's why when you find a label that fits you well, you'll probably want to stick with it.

The same holds true for various styles of clothes, some of which fit certain body types much better than others do. For example, while a woman with Rubenesque proportions may fit comfortably into a pair of size 8, pleated khakis from The Gap, the company's side-zip, flat front, more body-conscious version may not accommodate her fuller figure—no matter what size she tries. The bottom line: Once you have a handle on the MOs of enough designers and have zeroed in on the best style options for yourself, you'll meet with much greater success in finding clothing that fits just right.

Special Sizes

Are you one of the millions of men and women who don't have the "average" body that regular-size clothing is designed to fit? The following are for the growing minority who fall outside the norm (shorter or taller) than the average (5'4" woman or 5'11" man, or with larger proportions) that petite, short, tall, and women's (plus) sizes are made.

Fashion Footnote

Talk about cushioning the blow! As a rule, the more expensive the clothing, the smaller the size you need.

Fashion Footnote

Women's, or plus sizes are proportioned to fit those with fuller figures. Compared to regular misses sizes, women's sizes have a slightly lower bustline and a fuller cut.

Like other size charts, those for special sizes are best used as starting points for finding your correct size.

Petite Sizes

Size	2	4	6	8	10	12	14
	XS	XS	S	S	M	M	L
Bust	32	33	34	35	36	37 1/2	39
Waist	24	25	26	27	28	29 1/2	31
Hips	34	35	36	37	38	39 1/2	41

Women's Sizes

Size	14W	16W	18W	20W	22W	24W	26W
	1X	1X	2X	2X	3X	3X	4X
Bust	40	42	44	46	48	50	52
Waist	31	33	35	37	39	41	43
Hips	42	44	46	48	50	52	54

Big Men Sizes

Size	XXL	XXL	XXXL	XXXL
Neck	18	18 1/2	19	19 1/2
Chest	50	52	54	56
Waist	46	48	50	52
Hip	50 1/4	51 3/4	53 1/4	54 3/4

Fashion Footnote

Men's clothing is also sized according to height. In suits, you'll take a short if you're 5'3" to 5'7"; a regular if you're 5'8" to 5'10"; a long if you're 5'11" to 6'2"; an extra long if you're 6'3" to 6'7". For sportswear and outerwear, regular sizes fit men 5'8" to 5'10"; tall sizes fit those 5'11" to 6'3".

Creating a Better Fit

A host of design devices help make garments more flattering to the figure and/or more comfortable to wear. This brief overview will acquaint you with three of them.

Ease Up

A comfortable fit can rarely be had if a garment has too little wearing ease incorporated into it to accommodate. This fullness is a huge factor in how comfortable a garment will be, whether you're reaching across a desk or sitting through even a short meeting.

Wearing ease is provided through several design techniques, including pleats and gathers. *Pleats* are folds in the fabric that release to accommodate fullness; they are commonly seen in pants, on shirt backs, sleeves, and cuffs, and—to provide greater mobility—at the center back or side of a tightly fitted skirt. *Gathering,* a method in which a large amount of material is drawn into a smaller space, creates soft, even folds—usually at a waistband or shirt cuff.

The Fashion Police

If you buy clothing in a certain size mostly out of habit, take the time to try things on in a size bigger and a size smaller than normal. (There are over 21 sizes for men's suit jackets alone!) You may be surprised at how much better one of them fits.

The Fashion Police

When trying on clothing, don't just stand there: Squat, take a seat, reach for something. Unless you're employed as a guard at Buckingham Palace, you probably move around a lot at work and will want your clothes to fit comfortably.

As a rule, garments should incorporate at least 3 inches of wearing ease at the chest/ bust, 2 inches in the hips, and 1 inch at the waist. This is done at the design stage: An easy way to check is to measure around the waist of a pair of men's trousers. If they're supposed to be a 36-inch waist, they'll actually measure 37 or more inches.

The Art of the Dart

A *dart* is a pointed, V-shaped tuck sewn into a garment to help shape it to the curves and contours of the body. Usually found at the bust, shoulder, waist, and hips, a dart should point toward the fullest part of the contour to which it is conforming.

Shouldering the Burden

When properly positioned and sized, shoulder pads can simultaneously build up and even out weak or sloping shoulders, make hips looks slimmer, and cause you to look like you're standing more erectly. These are all good things. The problem arises, most commonly in womenswear, when designers either opt for too much of a good thing or choose pads that are the wrong size or shape for a garment. (Who isn't familiar with the effect of having two large lumps sitting atop the shoulders? Or the creation of fullback proportions?)

What you're looking for in shoulder padding is a very natural effect, just a bit bolder than what you were born with—think better, yet believable, proportion. The key is to find padding that covers the whole shoulder (bye-bye, lumps) and softly squares it off.

The Fashion Police

How many shoulder pads are too many? This is a common dilemma for women, since everything from blouses to jackets to coats are padded—often creating shoulders out to here! A good option is to remove the pads from tops that you frequently wear under jackets and to insert removable pads when you'll be wearing the shirt or blouse solo.

When is it safe to remove or replace shoulder pads that look too obvious? If they're accessible—that is, not buried underneath a lining—it's perfectly acceptable to detach the pads, especially if they're the removable kind. They, or a pair that's less bulky or more appropriately shaped, can always be reinserted later. For garments that are lined or tailored, seek the advice of a tailor (unless you're a skilled sewer); he or she will know how much change in padding a jacket can accommodate before the fit is compromised.

Good Fit: A Checklist

An honest-to-goodness good fit can be hard to find, but this checklist should make one easier to identify. You may want to take a copy with you when you hit the stores. The criteria here hold true for most traditional male and female business garb.

Jackets:

➤ The collar sits comfortably at the back of your neck, allowing about $^1/_4$ inch—and no more than $^1/_2$ inch—of the shirt collar to show.

➤ Shoulders fit squarely and extend no farther than about $^1/_2$ to $^3/_4$ inches from the edge of your shoulder.

➤ The jacket back lies flat against your shoulder blades.

➤ The bottom of the armhole doesn't dig into your armpits.

➤ It's long enough to completely cover your seat while you're standing.

➤ The sleeves hit the midpoint of the wrist bone, allowing about $^1/_2$ inch of your shirt cuff to show.

➤ The lapels lie flat, don't buckle or bunch, and don't pull open (a sign the jacket is too snug across the chest).

➤ The vents, the vertical slit(s) at the back or sides, lie flat and don't pull open.

➤ Buttons don't strain.

➤ The sleeves, shoulders, or jacket length don't require adjustment when you stand up.

Shirts:

➤ The collar gently hugs your neck. If you can get two or three fingers in around the neck when the shirt is buttoned, it fits.

➤ When arms are hanging naturally to the side, the sleeves reach the point where the wrist and hand meet.

➤ Sleeves are long enough—that is, slightly larger than your arms, and they can bend without pulling on the cuffs—so that they don't sneak up your wrists when you move your arms.

➤ Cuffs fit snugly, so that the sleeves won't fall over the hand.

➤ Armholes allow you to move your entire arm without consequence.

➤ Shoulder pads don't extend beyond the edge of the shoulder.

➤ Darts don't pucker.

➤ Buttons are securely anchored and well positioned so that there's no unintended exposure.

➤ Tails are long enough so that they won't pull out of your pants or skirt.

➤ The sleeves, collar, or shoulders don't require adjustment when you stand up.

Pants/Skirts*

➤ The waistband is on your waist and stays parallel to the ground all the way around you.* (The only exception: jeans, which usually ride lower.)

➤ You can insert two fingers into the waistband.

➤ Pleats lie flat when you're standing. If they spread too much, you need a size or two bigger.*

➤ Cuffs are in the neighborhood of 1$^1/_2$ inches high.

➤ The crotch neither rides up too high nor down too low.

➤ Your socks aren't visible when you're standing still or walking, unless it's due to the specific styling of the pants—for example, women's pants that taper at the ankle.

➤ Front creases should be symmetrical and cross the middle of your kneecaps.

➤ The garment falls straight from the hip.*

➤ Pockets stay closed.

➤ They don't ride up when you sit.*

➤ The leg reaches the top of your shoe on men, it then "breaks," or forms a short, horizontal crease, over the instep.

➤ Whatever length skirt you choose, the hem falls at the narrowest point of the leg—be it the calf, knee, or ankle. For longer lengths, that means it's either just above or below the widest part of your calf; if a shorter length is preferred, aim for a few inches above the knee*.

➤ Hems are even, never wavy.*

➤ The garment doesn't require adjustment when you stand up.*

* indicates information that's applicable to skirts

The Fashion Police

Vertical, horizontal, or diagonal wrinkling and puckering generally signal that a garment is either too small or too big.

A Perfect Fit: Alter-native Solutions

It would be folly to think that every garment you buy is going to fit you perfectly—with the incredible range in sizing variations almost nobody is an off-the-rack perfect fit. That's why practically everybody can use the services of a good tailor. Whether it's a simple fix (narrowing the lapels, letting out a pair of trousers) or a more complicated alteration (adding a slit to a skirt, shrinking too-big shoulders), making your clothes fit as well as possible is a worthwhile investment. (See Chapter 22, "Care And Keeping," for more information on alterations.)

The Least You Need to Know

➤ Nothing is more flattering than a good fit.

➤ Particularly for men, knowing your measurements is a good start to getting a good fit.

➤ Sizing varies from manufacturer to manufacturer, designer to designer. You may wear three different sizes from three separate lines.

➤ For a garment to fit just so, it needs to smoothly conform to the lines and curves of your body.

➤ Alterations are often necessary to provide a perfect fit.

Part 3
Building a Wardrobe

A real working wardrobe—that is, one that gets you through the week looking appropriately attired—doesn't just happen. For most people, it requires the thoughtful execution of a plan. And that's precisely how you can think of the next five chapters. Taken as a whole, they provide a complete course in the selection and purchase of clothing that will help you look like the success you know you can be.

In Chapter 7, "Getting Started," you'll find out how to evaluate what you already own, salvage the winners, and divest yourself of the poor performers. Then, in the next two chapters, you'll learn to select the clothing and accessories that best suit you and your work environment. After that, in Chapter 10, "So Many Options!," you'll discover the do's and don'ts of assembling a go-the-distance wardrobe and discover how to incorporate color and pattern into your wardrobe in a winning way.

Finally, in Chapter 11, "Milking Your Wardrobe for All It's Worth," you'll see firsthand how to "work" your wardrobe to get the most out of it. There, with the aid of photos and how-to tips, you're guaranteed to start thinking about your wardrobe more as a collection of pieces that mix and match and less as a closetful of individual items with limited potential.

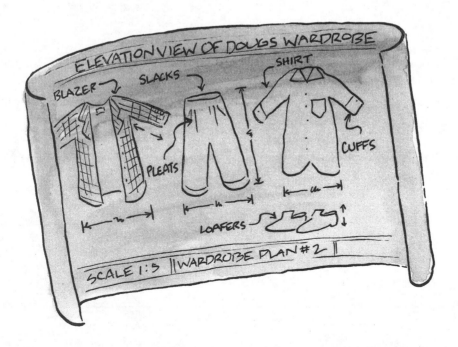

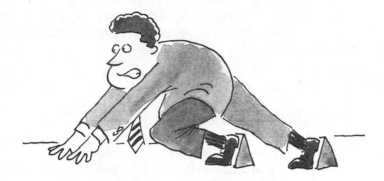

Getting Started

Put away that checkbook! Getting started doesn't mean making a beeline for the mall. Just as you wouldn't place an order for office supplies without checking how many Post-It Notes and staples were still on hand, you can't begin the task of building a solid working wardrobe without first taking inventory of what you already own and honestly evaluating the worth of each item. This project doesn't mean calculating an item's monetary value, but rather determining its ability to assist you in your drive to dress like the winner that you are.

Brace Yourself!

Make no mistake—this assessment of your apparel will require a certain measure of courage. Like pouring over your college photo album, weeding through your wardrobe will stir up some emotions—both good and bad. These clothes chronicle your professional and physical development over the years, including every job lost, every pound gained. Your search may turn up some clothing that you haven't even worn yet that nonetheless doesn't make the grade.

What should make this exercise less painful is the knowledge that, once the wheat is separated from the chaff, you'll be left with fewer clothes but less hassle. When you open your closet door, you won't have to see, and feel guilty about, those shoes that always pinched or the jacket with the puckering lapels. Instead, all you'll see is clothing that fits (and doesn't give you fits) and works for you (rather than against you). Sure, you'll probably need to fill in the gaps, but all in all, you'll wonder, why didn't I do this sooner? I promise.

Fashion Footnote

Are you one of the majority of women who fall into the decidedly female trap of turning such clothes encounters into opportunities to be critical of your body? Take a tip from the men and blame the garment and not your body when the former doesn't fit.

Ready, Set, Go

Since this kind of work can be tough on your ego, do it on a day when you're feeling good about yourself—that is, you're not two days into a diet, in dire need of a haircut, or maxed out on your credit cards. You'll also have to feel up to the assignment: Depending on the size of your closet and its chaos quotient, you'll need a big chunk of time—and a whole lot of stamina. Set aside a Saturday afternoon when you won't be disturbed and will be able to finish the job. Although wardrobe weeding won't be the most fun you've ever had, it is an important step toward cultivating a more polished, professional, and successful you!

The Fashion Police

It's a fashion felony to be without a full-length mirror. Pity the poor fellow who, without the help of a mirror, has neglected to zip his fly, or the woman who heads to the bus with her skirt tucked into the back of her hose. Taking a quick look in the full-length mirror should be the last thing you do on your way out the door—and don't forget the back view!

To start, you'll need a full-length mirror and a handheld one (for catching the rear view), good lighting (to see every bulge and line), four large boxes (label them *fix*, *archive*, *recycle*, and *toss*), and an objective eye. If, like many people, you don't have the latter (at least when it comes to how you look in your clothes), you may want to enlist the aid of someone whose opinion you trust and whose style you admire, and who isn't afraid to tell it to you straight—albeit in a kindly manner. ("Plaid pants, with your big butt?" is the kind of advice no one needs to hear.)

You'll want to think carefully about who to pick for this post. If you're a woman, a boyfriend or husband may not fit the bill. How to know? Determine from past experience if "it looks fine" is the extent of his evaluation skills. If you're a man, you'll probably prefer female support—a wife, girlfriend, sister, even your mother.

The Good, the Bad ... and the Ugly

Once you have everything—and everyone—assembled, it's time to get down to business. The goal is to try on every piece of clothing you own and determine whether it's a keeper or a clunker that's just taking up precious space and more than a few minutes of morning evaluation.

Why, you may be wondering, do I have to go through all my clothes when I'm just trying to establish a work wardrobe? Because, especially in this day of casual-business dressing, you may discover that a shirt or sweater designated as weekend wear can also go to work. Plus, if a business associate snags an extra ticket to a snazzy industry affair, won't you feel better accepting when you know that your black suit or dress still fits?

The Fashion Police

Believe it or not, there's even a "correct" way to dress while reviewing your wardrobe. Clean underwear and neutral-hued socks are musts for men; a smooth, supportive bra and sheer hose are in order for women. For those who easily become distracted by what's going on above the neck, applying some makeup and styling your hair may help you concentrate on the matter at hand.

The Review Process

Starting with your suits, and then moving on to the jackets and separates, divvy up your clothes into two categories: the ones that have worked for you time and time again and that make you feel good, and those that don't—and possibly never did. This task can be difficult, since having lots of clothes can give you a certain sense of security. Unfortunately, having a closet jam-packed with clothing you can't or won't wear isn't going to get you very far. So be ruthless. To make it easier, use this question-naire to determine each item's value:

➤ **Do you wear it?** If you consistently try on something and take it off, then you and it weren't meant to be. Not sure? The general rule of thumb is that if you haven't worn a garment in a year, you probably won't wear it again. (Of course, special circumstances do sometimes apply, as you'll see in a minute.)

➤ **Does it fit?** If a few nips and tucks are all it takes to remedy something (say, sleeves that are a smidgen too long), that's one thing. But if a garment feels uncomfortably tight (that is, it's 10 pounds too small, and weight loss isn't imminent), it'll only eat away at your self-esteem. Toss it. If you really can't bear to part with your "skinny" or "fat" clothes, set them aside and store separately.

➤ **How does it feel?** A fabric that doesn't breathe (for example, 100 percent acetate or polyester) can make you sweat, itchy fabrics only get itchier as the day wears on, and anything too stiff can compromise your creativity. The ultimate goal: A closet full of comfortable clothing.

➤ **Does it flatter?** Do turtlenecks emphasize your double chin? Does that cobalt blue shirt complement your coloring? (This is where that friend/spouse/sibling will come in handy.) After viewing yourself in the mirror, it should be an easy call to see if the item accentuates an asset or flaunts a flaw.

➤ **Is it in style?** A classic piece in a classic cut and color—say, an ivory cashmere crewneck, gray flannel trousers, or black suede loafers—is a keeper. (Here is where you can disregard the one-year rule.) If it's an article of clothing from a bygone era, you might want to say bye for good. While styles are cyclical (witness the recent resurgence of '70s clothing), chances are, when it comes around again, you will be too old to care or the style will have changed just enough to keep it looking dated.

➤ **Is it in good condition?** Some things just can't be fixed. Look for fabrics worn thin or shiny, permanently stained clothing, shoes that are just too run down. (See Chapter 22, "Care and Keeping," for tips on shoe repair.)

➤ **Does it smell funny?** It may sound strange, but the finishes applied to fabrics, say, to make them resistant to wrinkling, sometimes impart odors that can linger. I once found a very chic sweater set that had an odd, chemical odor. Thinking it just needed a good airing out, I bought it. The smell, however, never dissipated. As much as I love the twinset (and even though others don't notice the smell), I find myself avoiding it.

➤ **Is it appropriate for your job?** Is that navy blue suit too staid for the hip firm you're working at now? Are the boot-leg pants too trendy for a bank? Don't just think about your company's dress code, think also about the image you're trying to project. A word of caution: In this ever-changing job market, it's wise not to be too quick to deep-six your stuff. One friend jettisoned all of her conservative suits when she quit her job and went back to school. Imagine her regret when, just six months later, the same company lured her back.

Quote . . . Unquote

I base my fashion taste on what doesn't itch. ...Gilda Radner

➤ **Do you own more than one of these?** Safety in numbers may be a good rule for people, but having several of the same item—especially if just one of them really passes muster—is a psychological crutch. Remember: Now's the time to streamline. (I recently gave the boot to two of the three black cardigans I owned, keeping only the one I really like and frequently wear.) Otherwise (say, if having duplicates or triplicates is simply an indication of how much you like or liked something), refer back to the one-year rule.

After sorting through the large items, do the same with the things you don't hang up or keep in your closet: belts, scarves, sweaters, lingerie, skivvies, socks, and shoes. Just because these things take up less room doesn't mean they don't contribute to the clutter and confusion.

The Fashion Police

Ladies, when you're on the run, the last thing you need is a run in your pantyhose. Go through your entire stash, pitching those that can't be saved with nail polish. Keep in mind, too, that obvious repairs are no-nos for hose.

The Purge Process

By the time you've completed your review, you should have two piles—what works for work and what doesn't. Don't be discouraged if your toss pile towers over your keep pile; ultimately, it's a good sign—better to have fewer great options in your closet than too many wrong ones.

The next step: Starting with the discards, assign each to either the trash or recycle box. The trash box is a receptacle for those clothes that aren't fit for chum or charity. Unsalvageable items include ripped sweaters, jackets that are faded or worn thin at the elbows (or anywhere else for that matter), stained T-shirts and blouses, seriously scuffed or misshapen shoes.

The recycle bin is home to anything that you plan to give away. Into this box goes anything that, after careful consideration, just isn't going to work—even after a tailor gets his pins and needles on it. Don't feel guilty; for a friend, relative, or second-hand store, your old clothes are new. I just recently gave away a jacket I had hemmed and hawed over before buying five years ago; it was beautiful, but never, ever fit me right. Letting go after so many years of trying to wear it (I could only manage to once) was a truly liberating experience.

Dollars & Sense

If your discarded duds are in good condition, you can get cash for them from consignment shops. The Salvation Army, Goodwill, or women's shelters offer tax receipts. A third option: a "swap party," in which friends bring clothes they no longer want and trade with each other.

Jeepers, Keepers!

Those items that remain—the clothes that work—need to be separated as well. The three options are the archive or fix boxes and your closet. What goes where:

➤ **The archive box**—This box will hold the items you love but don't wear often, if ever (like vintage clothing or pieces with sentimental value). Those that mean most to you should be cleaned and stored in archival-quality garment bags or boxes, available in many specialty home stores.

➤ **The fix box**—In here goes anything that requires the attention of a tailor or dry-cleaner, including clothing that needs a button or cleaning, and those items that need to be shortened, let out, or overhauled. The latter is a tough call; you must decide whether you want to incur the cost of altering the jacket with the linebacker shoulders or cropping the pants that never felt right (see Chapter 22 for a price guide). If unsure, leave it there for the time being and return to this box when everything else is organized.

Fashion Footnote

Hey, guys! Whether it was a gift from your secretary or your mother, now is the time to muster your courage and toss any ties you really dislike (and while you're at it, chuck the clip-ons).

➤ **The closet**—The clothes that get returned to your closet should be grouped according to how often you wear them. Front and center are work clothes so that you have easy access in the a.m. Hard-core weekend wear (the stuff that doesn't even cut it on casual Fridays) takes a less prominent place in your closet, while out-of-season clothes should be hung to the side or the back. (See Chapter 22 for further detailing).

Put It in Writing

Taking inventory isn't finished until you make a written account of your assets. While this step may seem to be utterly ridiculous, it serves a useful purpose, namely, helping you in the future to make wise choices and avoid fashion fumbles. Face it: If the record indicates you already own three pairs of navy pants or black wing tips, you're less likely to buy another. On the other hand, a decided shortage of shirts can steer you to the right department.

Cataloging your closet isn't hard. Simply list—by season and category (pants, jackets, suits, shirts, accessories)—all the items that made the grade. Be specific in your detailing, especially if you own several like items. (Instead of noting that you own two gray sweaters, for example, indicate that one is a turtleneck and the other a polo style.) Keep this list at the ready for whenever the mall calls, which means in your wallet or purse if you're prone to spur-of-the-moment visits. For those who prefer visual reminders, a Polaroid is worth a thousand words.

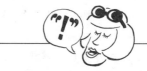

Quote . . . Unquote

List, Hamlet, list, O list! ... The ghost of Hamlet's father

Lessons Learned

Bravo! By now, your closet is neat and orderly, your drawers decluttered. But there's more to this exercise than seeing clear to the back of your closet. You should now have a much better understanding of your sartorial sense: which styles and colors appeal to you and which silhouettes work on you.

The opposite is also true: Discovering that beige washes you out, that cuffed trousers make you look shorter, and that you're now a size larger can be immensely helpful down the line. And, if nothing else, at least you're aware of your weakness for repeatedly buying garments in the same style or color. These are all good things to know before embarking on a shopping excursion.

The Least You Need to Know

➤ The first step toward creating a professional business wardrobe is determining what you already own.

➤ Each article of clothing needs to be evaluated individually and judged on its wearability.

➤ As hard as it may be to do, discarding any and all garments that don't make the cut makes it much easier to look your professional best.

➤ A written record of your wardrobe makes a handy reference when you're facing a mall full of stores, each filled with racks of clothing.

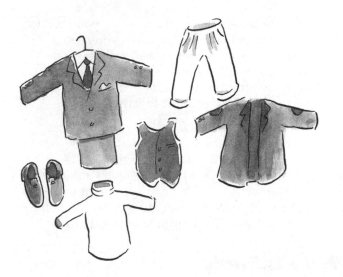

Chapter 8

The Basic Components

In This Chapter

➤ A suit to suit you

➤ Jacket options

➤ Tops and bottoms

➤ Dresses for success

Now that you've weeded out all the clothes that you don't (can't, won't, or—let's be honest—never did) wear, you'll need to restock. If you're thinking, "Yikes, it took me years to choose all those clothes that didn't work. How long is this going to take?"— fear not. This time around, you'll be operating with a new resolve, a fresh perspective, and a wealth of practical information that will help ensure quick success.

The first order of business is to learn the basics about the basics, the pants, jackets, shirts, skirts, and dresses that make up a go-the-distance working wardrobe. Once you have that down, the rest is easier.

A Suit of Clothes

Its styling will depend on everything from your profession to your physique, but the bottom line is that almost everyone needs the makings of a suit. It's a sizable investment, no doubt. But for those in all but the most casual environment, there's no

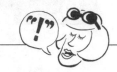

Quote . . . Unquote

The suit remains the uniform of official power. ...Anne Hollander, *Sex and Suits*

Fashion Footnote

Quality suiting fabrics are supple, resilient, and drape well, yet they typically have body—which gives substance and shape to even the most unstructured garment.

question it's the ensemble to turn to when you need to be "on," the sartorial solution for when you need to project poise, convey confidence, and make a good impression. Just what is it about a suit that affords it such impact? The unbroken line it creates simply makes you look like you've got your act together.

In addition to the positive subliminal messages that suits deliver, it's hard not to appreciate their ease. Suits help take the work—and much of the guesswork—out of dressing. It's so simple: One plus one equals an outfit. And for women, who often have the option of wearing either a skirt or pants with a matching jacket, one plus one plus one adds up to a multitude of possibilities.

What's Suitable

What kind of suit will work best for you? The traditional style is a somewhat stiff, sharply tailored two piece with classic lines and a formal bent—the late '90s version of the "power" suit. If you work in a conservative or corporate environment, it's the obvious—and sometimes only—choice. For those who toil in more relaxed business environments, the newer, less structured style—one that's still serious despite its softer edges—might be your best choice.

The real beauty of this new breed of relaxed businesswear is its versatility: When taken apart, the two (or three) pieces often work as separates, meaning the jacket pairs well with khakis, the pants with a twinset or denim shirt. (Skip ahead to Chapter 11, "Milking Your Wardrobe for All It's Worth," to see this principle put into action.) This flexibility isn't always the case with more traditional suits, especially men's, which are harder to separate and wear as individual parts.

No matter what style it is, if you're going to have just one suit (at least for now if you're just starting out), you'll want it to be made of wool or a wool blend. Whether woven into a gabardine or crepe, wool is by far the most versatile suiting fabric.

The Long and Short of Jackets

Without a doubt, jackets are the most pivotal elements of any wardrobe. Beside being the most expensive item you'll buy (short of a coat, that is), it's the one you can count on to lend presence, importance, and authority—even when dressing up a pair of khakis. (That's why the wisest workers will keep one handy in case of an unannounced visit from a board member or other bigwigs.

Whether you're buying one as part of a suit or to pair with other separates (the term used in the fashion industry to describe pants, skirts, and tops that coordinate, but don't necessarily match), jackets—especially women's—come in a wide variety of styles, and feature a number of design details. This overview will familiarize you with your options.

Staying Abreast

Men's jackets come in two styles: single- and double-breasted. For women, there's a third common option—jackets that button all the way up to the collar.

A single-breasted jacket is one that opens right down the middle, with buttons on one side of the opening, buttonholes on the other. Single-breasted jackets are the most flattering to a wide range of figure types and are the most versatile. The two-button, single-breasted suit is the most favored by men in the U.S., though it's not considered more correct than a three-button model.

Fashion Footnote

A man should choose a suit, which is cut in one of three silhouettes, according to his physique. The American, which is often called the sack suit, is the most conservative of the lot and the easiest to wear. It's single-breasted, boxy fashioned with little shoulder padding, and sports a single, centered vent. The Italian has a very snug fit and high, padded shoulders. The jackets are general ventless. This suit looks best on the slim and trim. The British adheres to the lines of the body, and has a nipped in waist and side vents. The shoulders are soft and lightly padded. Prince Charles wears this kind of suit.

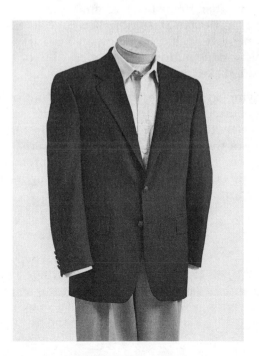

A single-breasted blazer, the cornerstone of many working wardrobes.

A double-breasted jacket usually has more verve than a single-breasted model.

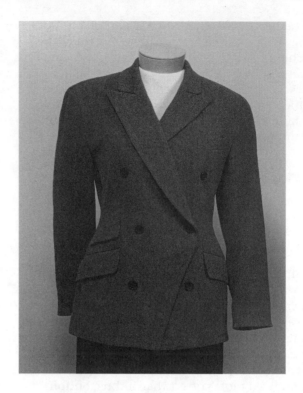

Double-breasted jackets, those that close by having one half of the front overlapping the other, have a bit more pizzazz than single-breasted models and usually look dressier. Double-breasted jackets have at least four, and as many as six, buttons; most are just for show. Only one working button is ever supposed to be buttoned, and it makes no difference which.

Staying on that issue, the appropriate buttoning of a two-button jacket is to close only the top button: if there are three buttons, you can close just the center one, or the top two. Choose the option that looks best on you. In case you're wondering the protocol, a jacket should be unbuttoned—but pulled straight—when you sit down.

Fashion Footnote

Men's jackets are said to unbutton on the left so that a right-handed man could reach his sword or gun more easily!

The Lowdown on Lapels

Wide or narrow, notched or peaked—these are the options you face when considering lapels. On single-breasted suits, the lapels are frequently notched, where a piece of fabric at the junction of the collar and the lapel looks as though it was snipped away. (A nonnotched, single-breasted exception: a woman's jacket with a shawl collar, which extends without interruption from the back of the neck down to the front closure.)

Double-breasted suits usually have wider peaked lapels, the type that jet out and form points. They're part of the aforementioned pizzazz.

Lapel width varies widely, from very thin to very broad, often according to the whims of fashion. While you'd do best to avoid either extreme, heftier men and women can carry off a somewhat wider lapel.

Pocket Picking

There are two types of jacket pockets, those that are completely visible on the outside of the garment, and those—called interior pockets—that have their inner workings hidden inside, between the good side of the jacket and the lining. There are three prevailing styles:

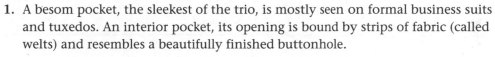

Dollars & Sense

Because trousers show signs of wear more quickly than jackets, it pays to buy two pairs of pants from the same dye lot (or a matching skirt) when purchasing a suit. That way, you're assured of having them when you need them.

1. A besom pocket, the sleekest of the trio, is mostly seen on formal business suits and tuxedos. An interior pocket, its opening is bound by strips of fabric (called welts) and resembles a beautifully finished buttonhole.

2. A flap pocket is probably the most common style. Though actually an interior pocket, the flap is on the exterior, covering the opening to the pocket. When placed on an angle, a flap is called a hacking pocket.

3. The patch pocket, the least formal and the type that holds the least, is sewn onto the outside of the jacket.

No matter what types of pockets your jacket has, keep in mind that when they're full the smooth draping of the fabric will be interrupted—so don't overstuff!

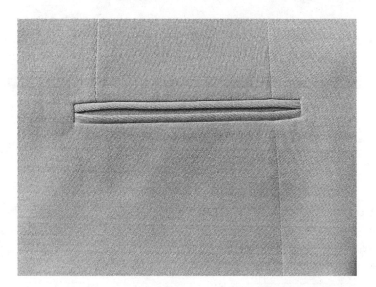

Besom pocket.

85

Flap pocket.

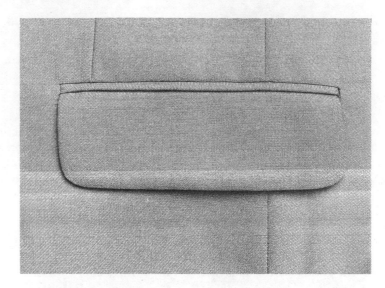

Patch pocket.

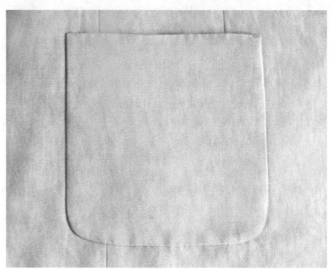

The Fashion Police

You know those little tags attached to the sleeve of new jackets or coats, the ones that inform you that the garment is made of 100 percent wool or has a Teflon finish? They should be (carefully!) snipped off before the garment is worn.

Cracker Jackets

If your office isn't a suit-and-tie kind of place every day of the week, there are less formal jacket options that allow you to look laid back, yet put together.

Fashion Footnote

The tailored suit can be traced all the way back to the linen padding meant to be worn under a suit of armor.

Good Sport

A *sport jacket* is simply a jacket without matching trousers. (The first sport jacket was commissioned by King George IV, who wanted it to wear while shooting on the estate of the Duke of Norfolk.) Though more casual than suit jackets, sport jackets can create any mood, depending on the fabric—everything from suede to tweed, linen to corduroy.

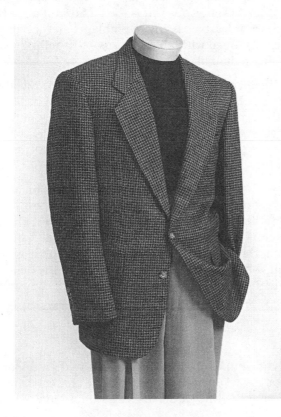

Sport jackets, like this one in a houndstooth check, offer the casual elegance that's ideal for dress-down Fridays. (Jacket courtesy of AKA Eddie Bauer.)

Ideally, sport jackets are real wardrobe extenders; the key is to carefully choose one to work with several pairs of pants and/or skirts. Again, the most versatile is a single-breasted model in a classic jacket style. Don't think, however, that a solid color is necessarily your only option: A sport jacket in a snappy herringbone or subtle tweed may be just the ticket if most of your bottoms are solids.

Though the term sport jacket is exclusive to menswear, for women, too, the un-matched jacket is a wardrobe mainstay. Unlike the male versions, women's jackets come in a range of styles—including boleros, peplums, top-of the-hip, and waist-length. When versatility is the main object, stick to the classic, below-the-hip style—which provides the most mileage.

What in Blazers ...?

Though technically a sport jacket, a blazer plays such a key role in our work wardrobes that it deserves to be separated from the pack. So, how exactly does a blazer differ from a sport jacket? This can be a tricky question to answer, since many people refer to any jacket that's not part of a suit as a blazer.

Fashion Footnote

Vests, which come in a wide variety of fabrics and styles, can often stand in for a jacket—especially when they're cut from traditional suiting material, like tweed and flannel.

Traditionally, whether single- or double-breasted, a blazer is black or blue and made of a medium-weight fabric. Making it even more distinguishable from other jackets, however, is the fact that it also still bears at least a passing resemblance—especially when emblazoned with gold buttons—to a military jacket, the original blazer.

The blazer made its debut on the British Naval frigate, the H.M.S. blazer, in the 1820's. Legend has it that the captain of the ship outfitted his crew in navy blue jackets with brass buttons in honor of the coronation of Queen Victoria, who immediately made it the official uniform of her fleet.

Through the years, as blazers become associated with yachting, they took on an air of elitism. Wearing a blazer these days, however, is a sign of how smart you are—not how snobby. That's because they're versatile, looking equally correct with jeans, khakis, and dressy pants. In fact, wearing one with, well, just about anything, will gain you instant respectability. Keep in mind, though that unless you want to look like the captain of a ship, you'll sport a single-breasted style without a crest on the breast pocket. Think twice, too, about whether you want brass buttons, which can limit the jacket's versatility.

Softer Stand-Ins

If you think all jackets have to be cut from cloth, think again—knitted pieces are ideal substitutes for more structured, woven jackets. They're also off the charts when it comes to comfort. But alas, only one style—the cardigan—is good for guys.

Cardigans. A button-down-the-front sweater named for the Earl of Cardigan, who led the Charge of the Light Brigade, cardigans work best at work for women when they're long and on the slim side, for men when they're worn with a tie, and for both genders in patterns and colors that scream establishment. Women in particular shouldn't underestimate a cardigan's versatility: When belted over a crisp, white shirt, a cardigan is a good mate for flannel trousers as well as jeans.

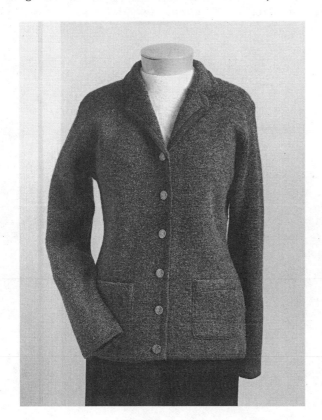

A cardigan is a fine stand-in for a jacket. (Cardigan courtesy of JCPenney.)

The Fashion Police

One caveat about women's sweater dressing, particularly in conservative and/or male-oriented cultures: When you're wearing a sweater that's fuzzy, fussy, or fluffy—especially if it's in a pretty pastel—you run the risk of being taken less seriously. Better bets are flat knits and classic cables in authoritative colors.

Twinsets. The components of the twinset, a cardigan and a matching pullover, not only combine to create a very in-charge effect for women, both also work on their own. Wear one to soften up a pair of pinstriped pants or dress up a pair of khakis.

Knit Jackets. They're as close as you'll get to the real thing, just a little less uptight. In very conservative environments, however, the most tailored examples—especially when paired with a matching skirt—may be too overtly sexual. Boxier or more loosely fitting styles are safest.

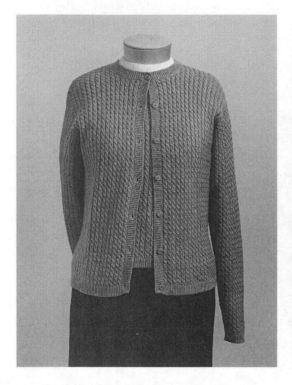

A cable-knit twinset dresses up khakis, softens a suit.

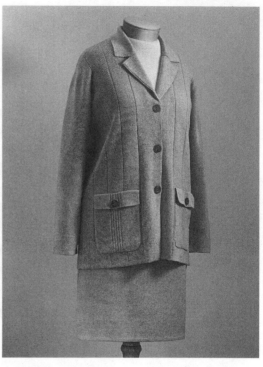

A knit jacket with matching skirt is a relaxed alternative to a tailored suit.

Fashion Footnote

Regardless of what jacket style you opt to buy, don't forget what you'll wear under it. If you like to layer a lot, consider buying a larger size or a roomier style.

Top Notch

Especially when you're just starting out, and don't have a closetful of clothes to work with, what you wear on top has the ability to keep the same old pieces below looking fresh and new. Luckily, shirts and sweaters are usually the most affordable acquisitions you can make. They're also part of a clothing category that's loaded with options, which are outlined here.

The Shirt Story

How important are shirts? Think about it: While you may frequently remove your jacket at work (if you even wear one at all), how often are you without your shirt? Hopefully not very, which makes them very important.

Fabric. As dress codes have loosened up, shirts for work have become acceptable in a wide range of fabrics, colors, and patterns. In the most conservative arenas, though, traditional shirting fabrics (like oxford cloth and broadcloth) in blue and white—or blue-and-white striped—are still the ticket for men. Women, however, have a bit more leeway, including softer, drapier silks and silk-like fabrics.

The Fashion Police

Should you monogram your shirts? Once considered a touch of class, monograms are now often thought to be too flashy and a mark of insecurity. "Who cares what your initials are? You should speak for yourself or your clothes should speak for your good taste," says one executive.

Fit. Ideally, the fit of a shirt should correspond to the tailoring of what's going over it, meaning that a more structured jacket calls for a more fitted (or tapered) shirt, and vice versa. A side benefit of a tapered shirt: Without all that excess fabric, it'll tuck into your trousers more easily.

Collars. On both men and women's dress shirts, a rolled collar is the preferred choice. This kind of collar first stands up from the neck edge and then falls down to rest on the garment. Within this category of collar, there are several variations, many of which give a shirt its name.

➤ **Button-down**—A collar that is secured to the shirt by two small buttons at the collar points, to keep it held neatly in place (The button-down was originally designed to keep shirt collars from flapping up in the faces of galloping polo riders.) The least dressy collar type looks swell with sport jackets. When worn with a tie, be sure that the knot isn't so thick that it strains the collar points. Worn open, it doesn't require a tie. If you like the effect of a button-down collar, but not the look, considered the new alternative—a button-down shirt that has the buttons hidden underneath the collar. A number of manufacturers now offer them.

➤ **Convertible**—A collar that can be worn open or fastened by a small, concealed button and loop. When closed, a convertible collar resembles a spread or straight collar.

Fashion Footnote

The one shirt everyone should own: a plain, white cotton shirt. Its versatility is unparalleled, looking—as it does—equally great with jeans and pinstripes, pearls or a tie, on its own or paired with a T-shirt or a blazer. Guess it isn't called a classic for nothing.

➤ **Shawl**—A collar and lapel that curve seamlessly from the back of the neck down to the front closure; it's most common on women's shirts.

➤ **Spread**—A collar that's spread wider apart than regular types. A more formal style, it should always be worn with a tie. The British spread has an even wider distance between the points, making it that much more formal.

➤ **Straight**—Also called the point collar, this collar is the most common of all. The length of the points vary and point downward.

➤ **Tab**—Strictly a man's shirt, since it features two small tabs that prop up a tie and hold it securely in place. The tabs are hidden from view once the tie is tied.

Gaining in popularity is the banded collar, which is basically a shirt without a collar. In olden days, separate shirt collars used to attach to this band of fabric, but now it's considered fashionable to go without. If dressing for an occasion where a tie is a must, a banded-collar shirt is a don't, since it doesn't accommodate a tie.

Shirt collars (clockwise from top): Button-down, tab, spread, shawl, banded, convertible, straight.

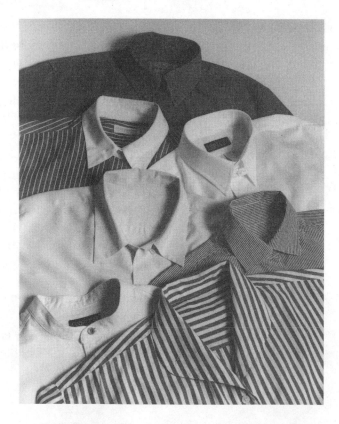

Cuffs. Shirts can have one of two types of cuffs, French or barrel. French cuffs, the dressiest kind, fold over on themselves and usually demand cuff links. Barrel cuffs, the more common type, close with a button or two.

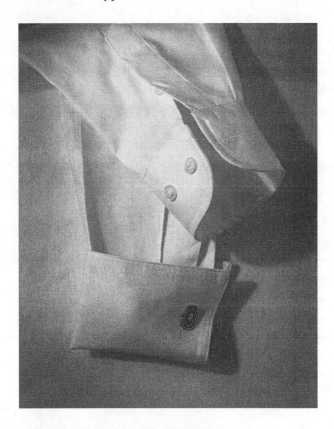

Shirt cuffs: Barrel cuffs (top) close with a button; the more elegant French cuffs require cuff links. (Cuff links courtesy of Lands' End.)

The Shirts on Your Back

Shirts for work can take many forms, other than the traditional type worn with suits and ties. Here's a rundown:

➤ **Polo shirt**—Originally a shirt worn to play polo (hence its name), this pullover with a rolled collar and anywhere from one to four buttons at the neck looks equally stylish under a blazer or atop khakis. At its least casual, it has long sleeves.

➤ **Camp shirt**—Distinguished by two patch or flap pockets and a notched collar, camp shirts can look sporty (especially short-sleeve styles) or positively elegant in more luxurious silk and linen.

➤ **T-shirt**—A huge category unto themselves, T-shirts can be long or short-sleeved; round-, square-, V-, or boat-necked; pocketed or plain; striped or solid; and knitted in everything from cotton to cashmere.

The Fashion Police

The right collar can help flatter a less than perfectly shaped face. The rule of thumb: Wear collars that aren't shaped the same way as your face! For example, someone with a long face shouldn't wear a straight collar with lengthy points (which would drag his or her face down further), while someone with a round kisser should (to give it more length).

The Sweater Set

Whether layered under suits or standing alone on casual days, sweaters are as indispensable as good assistants. In general, the hardest working are the following five: work suitability depends on a sweater's weight or ply, with finer-gauge knits getting the nod for dressier assignments.

Crewneck. A round-necked pullover style, crewnecks look best worn under sport jackets, or solo when no jacket is required. When worn over a collared shirt, the collar goes inside the sweater. Avoid at work: Anything big and bulky or would look at home around the campfire.

Polo. A sweater version of the polo shirt, it's the essence of casual elegance when buttoned all the way up (and worn under a jacket in place of a shirt), or left open with a T-shirt underneath—for a sportier effect.

Tunic. A thigh-length pullover that usually falls straight from the shoulder. When paired with a matching straight skirt or slim pants, it looks sleek and serious (so long as isn't tight around the hips or buttocks).

Turtleneck. Turtlenecks, which have high necks (about 5-inches worth), are good stand-ins for shirts when worn under all but the most tailored of suits. If your neck doesn't like feeling crowded, fold the turtle in half, or try a mock turtle, which is a shorter version of the full-fledged model.

V Neck. Of all the sweaters with a V-shaped neckline, only those that plunge the least work at work without something underneath. Sleeveless styles keep jacket sleeves from getting cramped.

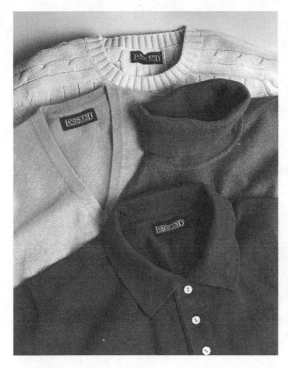

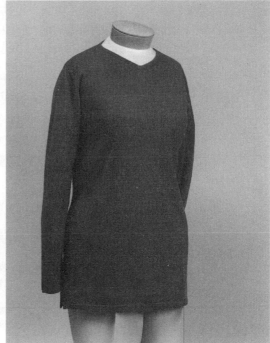

Sweater styles (from top): Crewneck, V-neck, turtleneck, polo.

Tunic sweater.

The Bottom Line

As in all fashion matters, men have fewer choices than women—who can choose between pants and skirts.

One Leg at a Time

Slacks are the pant version of sport jackets, the unmatched trousers that pair with other separates. There's not that much variation in trouser styling for men, save for the fabric. The biggest issues are pleats and cuffs.

Pleats. Pleats come in several varieties: single-, double-, or triple-forward (which open toward the zipper), single-, double-, or triple-reverse (which open toward the pockets), and box (which look like rectangular folds of fabric). Double and triple pleats are slightly dressier, and the straighter lines created by forward pleats are considered to be more conservative.

Whether to choose pants with or without pleats is your preference, but they do have some important aesthetic and functional benefits. For example:

➤ Pleats anchor the line of the pants, allowing them to fall better when something—like hands or change—is in pockets.

➤ Pleats permit more fullness in the thighs, knees, and derriére, and make sitting more comfortable.

Flat-front pants, which have little extra bulk, are more slimming—a good option if you have something to hide.

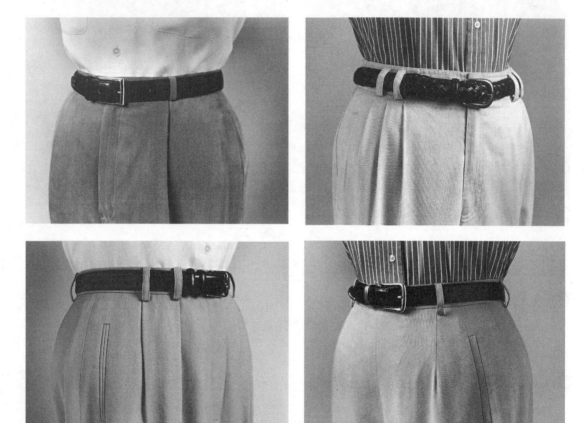

As you pleats (clockwise from top left): Single-reverse pleats, triple-reverse pleats, flat-front pants, box pleats.

Cuffs. Like pleats, the decision to cuff or not cuff is strictly a personal one. Some factors to weigh:

➤ Cuffs visually shorten the leg by breaking the vertical line, so you may want to go cuffless if your legs are on the short side. (Women can compensate by wearing heels, which elongate the leg.)

➤ Cuffs add weight to the bottom of the pants, which helps keep creases running straight down.

➤ Cuffs provide an elegant finish that makes a pair of trousers look more costly.

Women have more variety when choosing pants, but a close approximation of the classic, tailored pant will provide the most mileage—be it in a fuller cut with a wider leg (to better fit fuller figures) or a slimmer cut with straighter legs (for trimmer physiques). Unless you're in the market for something trendy to energize your wardrobe, avoid exaggerated styling—too-high or -low waistbands or legs that are too wide, flared, or narrow. Pleats and cuffs are just as common in women's pants, and the same factors apply when deciding whether to go with or without.

Fashion Footnote

Khakis, which are named—in honor of their original olive-drab color—for the Hindu word for dirt, have come full circle: from military-uniform fabric to an integral part of the work uniform. Made of a hardworking, smooth 100-percent cotton twill, khakis are often referred to as *chinos*.

Skirting the Issue

For women in conservative organizations, skirts are often a must. But even if pants are permitted, there will still be occasions when a skirt is the only option. That means everybody needs at least one. What follows is a report on the most work-appropriate styles. Whichever ones you choose, know that, when possible, a skirt should be lined. Not only will it fit better, it won't be see-through and will help serve you modesty-wise.

Straight. The straight skirt, a classic style that skims your waist and hips, is an essential you can wear with almost everything. Whether long or short, it creates a slim silhouette underneath a jacket. The key to this skirt is its fit. That's why many styles come in both a roomier, pleated-front style and a flat-front version. Some variations on the same theme: Trumpet skirts are straight skirts that start flaring out about two-thirds of the way down; pencil skirts, which are straight skirts in the extreme, are quite possibly too tight for many offices.

A-Line. Of all the silhouettes, the A-line, which gets wider as it gets longer, receives an A-plus for flattering those with heavier legs and fuller hips. To avoid looking shapeless, team A-line skirts with jackets with defined waists. The best fabric for an A-line skirt is something drapey;

Fashion Footnote

It's not a crime to buy multiples of something you really love.

in anything too stiff or heavy, the skirt looks as if it could stand up by itself.

Wrap. A wrap skirt is a style within a style. Both straight and A-line skirts can be designed to wrap around the body and fasten with one or more button or ties. Those that button close provide a more streamlined effect.

Pleated. Pleats add visual interest to a garment and, depending on the style, can alternately help flatter a figure, or emphasize a figure flaw.

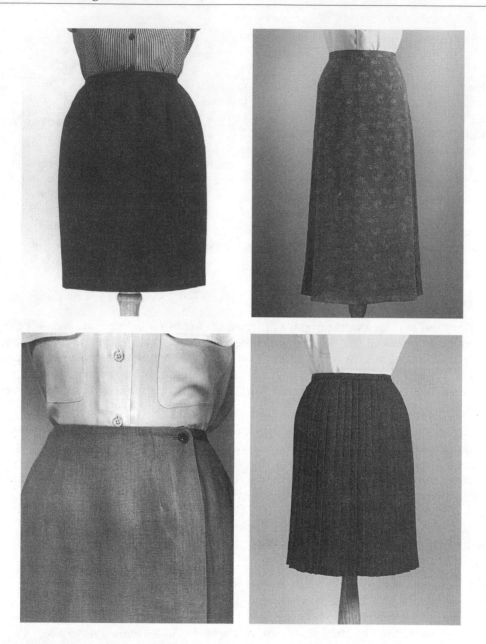

Skirt styles (clockwise from top left): Straight skirt, A-line skirt (courtesy of Liz Claiborne Collection), knife-pleated skirt, wrap skirt (courtesy of Eddie Bauer).

Best Dressed

A piece of clothing that requires no matching, no thought, no time—just pull it on and go. That perfectly describes a dress, the essence of time-management dressing.

For the longest time, women thought that dresses were too feminine to make it in the rough-and-tumble business world. And certain styles—namely slip, sun, and strapless—definitely are. But these days, some women's wardrobes revolve exclusively around dresses. That's because a number of styles work beautifully on the job.

Coat Dress. What could be more appropriate for work than a dress that's virtually a very long blazer? The coat dress, a classic since the '30s, is probably the most conservative dress style. Yet because it usually has a well-defined waist, a coat dress whispers femininity. They're particularly commanding in dark colors and fabrics with body.

Shirtwaist. The key to shirtwaist dresses is choosing a slim, tailored style that looks more like a dress with shirt styling than a shirt trying to pass as a dress. Work-worthy fabrics run the gamut from the sturdy to the more drapey.

Sheath. A sheath, which has the ability to make every woman look as though she has an hourglass figure, is most effective at work when worn under a matching jacket. A close, less work-appropriate cousin of the sheath is the shift, which has an A-line shape and no defined waist—so the fabric hangs away from the body.

The Fashion Police

Don't slip up: When you're wearing a skirt or dress that can become see-through when the light shines through it, you need a slip.

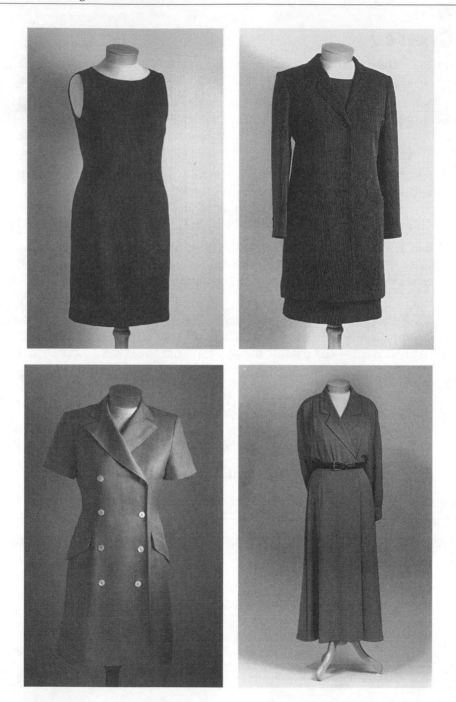

One-stop dressing (clockwise from top left): Herringbone sheath (courtesy of Liz Claiborne Collection), sheath with matching jacket, coatdress, shirtwaist dress.

The Least You Need to Know

➤ Some semblance of a suit, be it a more traditionally tailored style or one that's less structured, is a must for most people in the workforce.

➤ If yours is a relaxed work environment or you dress casually on occasion, a selection of mix-and-match jackets, pants, and skirts can provide considerable mileage.

➤ A white cotton shirt and dark wool blazer are essential items for your working wardrobe.

➤ Dresses are appropriate on the job, and they're the easy answer for women on tight schedules.

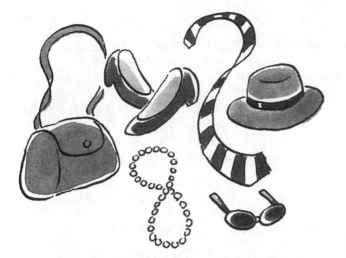

Chapter 9

Accessories: Special Effects

In This Chapter

➤ Notes on neckwear

➤ Silver and gold: jewelry on the job

➤ Keeping watch

➤ On specs

➤ Footnotes: shoes and socks

➤ Leatherworks: belts, handbags, briefcases

Accessories may be the smallest items in a work wardrobe, but they can pack a big punch, often creating the distinction between being just dressed and being dressed for success. Carefully chosen, these essential extras can pull together any look, adding polish and panache—and at least a hint of the personality of the wearer—to even the plainest basics.

At their most versatile, accessories can change the entire tone of an outfit, rendering it more relaxed or more formal, sporty or sophisticated, yet still perfectly fitting for the office. But the best part? Without having to cost a bundle themselves, these small additions still manage to make moderately priced suits and separates look far more expensive.

The key is investing in elegant, stylish accessories that give your look a well-deserved promotion. Up next, a rundown on the accessories that will complete your work wardrobe, followed by some words of wisdom on wearing them to best effect.

Fit to Be Tied

It's certainly not the reason a tie is called a tie, but there's no doubt that these long, thin strips of fabric can tie together a man's entire outfit. Even though it's often perfectly appropriate to go without (and even considered hip when the shirt is buttoned up all the way), a jacket and shirt simply look more finished when topped off with a tie. (That a new tie can also make the shirt and jacket duo look radically different confirms its standing as the champion wardrobe extender.)

But there's much more to ties than their ability to complete and change a look. They're the hallmarks of a guy's personal style, one of the simplest and least expensive ways for him to express his individuality.

Of all the accessories, however, none is being more affected by the loosening of dress codes than the necktie. But that doesn't mean banishing the lot of them to the back of your closet; there's no rule that says you can't wear a tie with khakis. In fact, you may want to continue taking advantage of the respectability and professionalism a tie affords. (It couldn't hurt!)

How many ties a man owns is up to him. Even if he has to wear one everyday, he may be content with just four or five (life's already filled with enough decisions, so why complicate matters?). Other guys need one in every color and every pattern. "It's practically the only way we have to set ourselves apart," laments one businessman. However many you need (and for the record, no one—no matter how casual his job—should have just one), here are some guidelines for choosing them:

➤ Coordinate a tie with the rest of your outfit. The easiest way is by picking one color in your ensemble to match it to.

➤ Pick ties that suit your personality. That said, shun silly, splashy, or goofy-looking ties. The novelty fades fast, but the memory of you wearing one may remain.

➤ Buy ties made of natural fibers: Silk is the most elegant and produces the best looking knots with the least amount of effort, but cotton is ideal for summer and casual wear. And so long as they're lightweight, wool ties are fine in colder weather.

➤ Wear wider ties with wider jacket lapels, and thinner ties with thinner lapels.

➤ Make sure the tie is long enough. It should reach your belt, with the narrow end (the tail) even with or

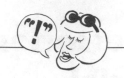

Quote . . . Unquote

Our ability to accessorize is what separates us from the animals. *...Steel Magnolias*

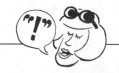

Quote . . . Unquote

Would it have killed you to put on a tie? *...David Letterman* a tad bit shorter than the wide end (the apron). There's no regulation length for ties (they range from about 52 to 58 inches, so—especially if you're tall—either tie it before you buy it to be certain, or bring along one of your own that's the right length to measure against. You may also want to check out the display of extra-long ties found in may stores.

How to Buy a Tie

A well-made tie will meet a certain criteria. Here's what to look for:

➤ The lining can be full length or partial, but should extend to the tips of the tie.

➤ Ties should have a full-length interlining that feels firm. This wool or canvas strip helps prevent wrinkling.

➤ The folds in the back of the tie should be loosely stitched together to help make the tie lie flat.

➤ At either end, there should be a horizontal bar of stitches tacking together the folds.

➤ A tie should have "body," and shouldn't be pressed flat.

➤ When held over your hand, the narrow end of a tie should fall directly in the middle of the wide end—no corkscrewing to the left or right. If it doesn't hang straight, it will never lie flat.

➤ Handstiching is a mark of quality tailoring.

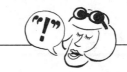

Quote . . . Unquote

A well-tied tie is the first serious step in life. ...Oscar Wilde

Tying the Knot

You can't wear a tie without knowing your knots, or at least knowing your preference among the Windsor, the half-Windsor, and the four-in-hand.

➤ The Windsor is the thickest knot in the bunch. It's named for the Duke of Windsor, who wore it to complement his wide, spread collars. The downside: It's bulky and, because of all the twists and turns it takes, requires a long tie.

➤ The half-Windsor is a Windsor that's been downsized. Wear it with a spread or straight collar.

➤ The four-in-hand is a small, straight knot that can be adjusted to fit any collar style.

Four-in-hand knot:
*Begin with the wide end of
the tie hanging down on
your right, about a foot
below the narrow end.
Cross the wide end over,
and then back under, the
narrow end. Bring the wide
end across again and then
up through the neck loop.
Hold the knot loosely in
place while passing the
wide end down through it.
To cinch, hold the narrow
end and slide the knot up
to the collar.*

Four-In-Hand

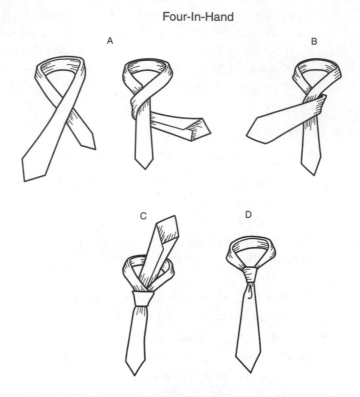

Half-Windsor knot: *Start
with the wide end of the
tie hanging down on your
right, about a foot below
the narrow end. Cross the
wide end over, and then
back under, the narrow
end. Bring the wide end up
through the neck loop, and
then pass it around the
front from left to right.
Feed the wide end up
through the neck loop and
down through the knot. To
tighten the knot, hold it
while gently pulling down
on the wide end. Then,
holding the narrow end,
slide the knot up to the
collar.*

Half-Windsor

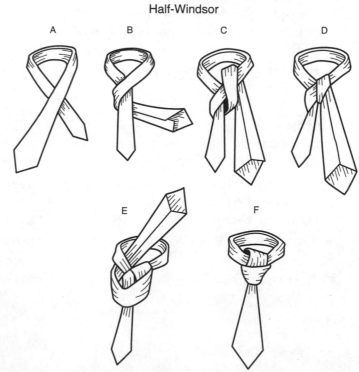

Take a Bow

Few sartorial issues provoke more heated debate than that of the bow tie, and those in favor are almost always in the minority. "They're not modern," "they're an affectation," and "they make you look arrogant (or like a buffoon, stuffed shirt, Orville Redenbacher)," are just a few of the comments collected from an informal survey.

But perhaps you're the exception, the guy—who, like FDR and Churchill—looks worldly and wise in a bow tie. To be sure, get some feedback before venturing out—or at least to anywhere very important. (One lawyer checks his calendar before tying one on, at the risk of turning off clients who wouldn't see them as the novelty he does.) If the ayes have it, bow on.

Fashion Footnote

A tie is well tied if it has a slight dimple in the middle, just below the knot. To achieve, neatly pinch the fabric directly underneath the knot after you've tied the tie but before tightening the tie up to your throat.

Bow Tie

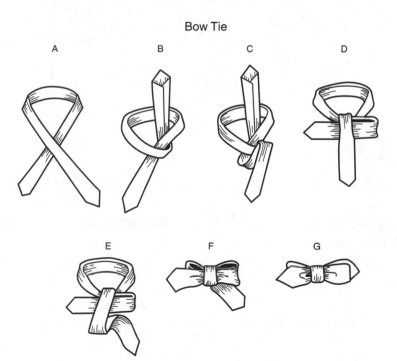

Bow tie: (Don't be nervous, it's like tying a shoelace—just around your neck!) Start with the left end 1" below the right. Tie the long end over and up behind the short one. Fashion a loop with the short end, centering it where the knot will be, and bring the long end over it. Form a loop in the long end and poke it back through the center, forming a knot. Adjust the ends slowly to tighten the knot.

Fashion Footnote

Ties are a distant relative of cravats, which were first worn by warriors on French battlefields in the 17th century.

Pocket Panache

An optional accessory that adds a certain flair to both men's and women's attire, the pocket square gets its name from the fact that it's made up of a square piece of fabric. (Don't think you have to buy an expensive model; a remnant from the fabric store works quite nicely.)

There are a number of different ways to fold one. With this version, the puffed method, it looks as though you casually stuffed the breast pocket (though achieving that effect requires some practice), rather than attempting a more formal, studied result.

Pocket square: Pick up a flattened square in the center. Holding the square with one hand about two-thirds of the way down, fold it so that the center of the square is a bit longer. Place the square in the pocket, and arrange/neaten as needed.

Pocket Square

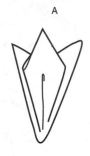

A

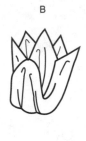

B

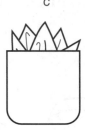

C

A few pointers on pocket squares:

➤ They shouldn't match your tie, but rather should coordinate with it, picking up a color.

➤ A tie and pocket square should be fashioned of contrasting fabrics. For instance, if you're wearing a silk tie, go with a linen or cotton square.

➤ They should stick out only about 1 to $1^1/2$ inches.

➤ A plain cotton handkerchief doubles quite nicely as a pocket square.

➤ Only in an emergency should you use your pocket square to blow you nose or mop you brow—that's what your handkerchief is for.

Scarves: Tie One on

Neckwear is an equal-opportunity accessory: Just as men have ties to update, excite, and expand their wardrobes, women have scarves. The secret to wearing them well is to achieve an unstudied effect, one that's not too fussy and doesn't look as though you tried too hard. (As with the pocket square, achieving such casual perfection takes practice!)

When choosing scarves, consider what effect you want them to create. A small cotton square can dress down whatever it's worn with, while a silk scarf will dress up denim. A colorful scarf can brighten up a dark jacket, while a cream-colored chiffon scarf will soften a sober beige suit. The combinations are as varied as your imagination.

How many scarves do you need? Start with a small wardrobe of prints and solids; so as not to limit yourself, include a handkerchief-size square, an oblong, and a larger square that's not too oversized (36 inches is a good size). Silk, chiffon, and cotton are good fabrics to build a wardrobe around.

Once you have them, what should you do with your scarves? There are probably a hundred ways to tie a scarf. Below are instructions for five of the most classic, all of which are appropriate in even the most conservative offices.

Hacking Knot

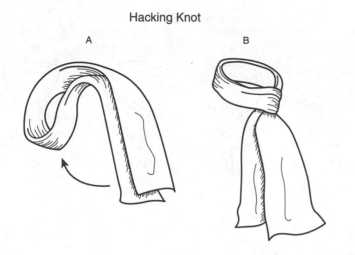

A   *B*

Hacking knot: *Double an oblong scarf and wrap it around the neck. Insert ends into the loop, and pull back in the opposite direction until scarf fits as snugly as desired.*

Knotted Neck Wrap

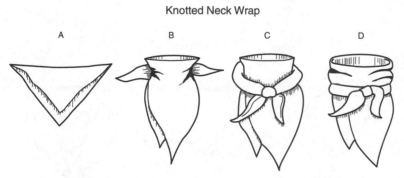

A   *B*   *C*   *D*

Knotted neck wrap: *Fold a square scarf into a triangle, placing the point in the front. Cross the ends at the back of the neck, bring them forward, and tie into a square knot over the front of the scarf. Tuck into collar or leave out.*

109

Feminine ascot: Lay a square scarf on a flat surface, wrong side up. Pick it up, and tie a knot at the center. Fold the scarf into a triangle with knot on the inside, place around the neck (with triangle in front), and tie opposite corners at the back of the neck. Tuck triangle into collar.

Feminine Ascot

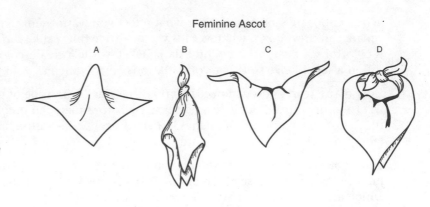

A   B   C   D

Neckerchief square knot: Fold a square scarf into an oblong shape and place it around the neck, keeping the right end about 2" longer than the left. Cross the long end over the short one and feed up through the neck, creating a single knot. Cross the long end, which is now on the left side, over the short end and feed it through the opening from behind. Pull ends to tighten. Wear knot in front or to the side.

Neckerchief Square Knot

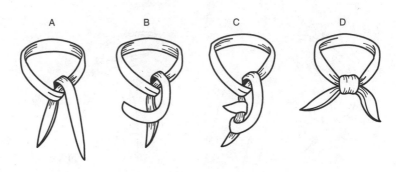

A   B   C   D

Granny knot: Fold a square scarf into a triangle, and place around the neck, keeping the ends even. To tie a granny knot, flip the ends over the top of the scarf, and feed them through the newly created loop from the back to the front. Pull the ends to tighten.

Granny Knot

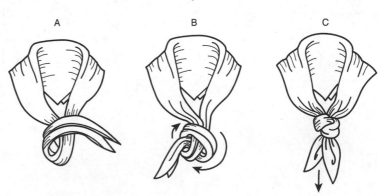

A   B   C

The Best of Times

Everyone needs a watch, whether it's to determine how many hours 'til quitting or lunch time, or if you're late for a meeting. But not just any watch will do. Unless your position requires you to keep track of split times or water pressure, the watch you want for work is a classic timepiece, one with moveable hands and numbers. Whether it's gold or silver, a Rolex or a Timex is a personal matter, as is whether you require the precision of a quartz movement. Just aim for elegant, or—if your dress code is more casual—elegant and sporty (and no, the two aren't mutually exclusive).

Fashion Footnote

Scarves and ties are handy ways to divert attention to the face and away from trouble spots below the neck.

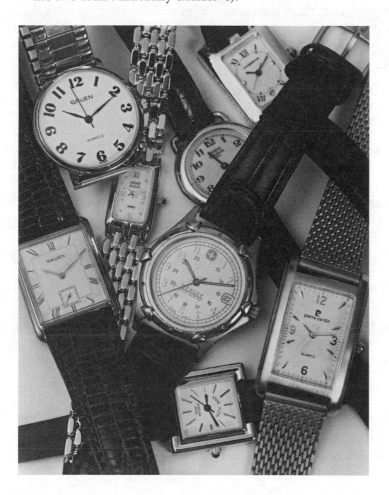

Keep time with an elegant watch.

Fashion Footnote

Quartz watches are extremely accurate, varying only about one minute each year.

Business Baubles

There are two words to describe the jewelry you should wear to work: simple and tasteful. As a rule, even the most casual office isn't the place to display an armful of plastic bracelets, a gaudy pinkie ring, or earrings shaped like palm trees. It is, however, your opportunity to quietly express your personal style.

His

Men aren't allowed much adornment, at least from nine to five. Cuff links are one of the tiny bits of glimmer they're permitted to wear in the office, and anything from gold ovals to fabric knots to slightly more whimsical styles will work—i.e., a pair that reflects your hobby or profession. Also acceptable are wedding and conservative rings, like signets and college rings. Collar pins and tie clips are your call (they're reportedly fading in popularity), but bracelets and necklaces are pushing the envelope.

The Fashion Police

Pull out a leaky Bic when a client asks if you've got a pen, and your professional image will surely suffer. Better to have on hand a slim, expensive-looking writing instrument—which can be purchased for under $10 at stationery stores.

Hers

Always right are the classics: pearl earrings, diamond studs, a drop earring in a semiprecious stone, smallish hoops, link and chain necklaces and bracelets, a single or multiple strands of pearls, a choker of sterling silver beads, a faux tortoise cuff or bangle, an antique-y pin or heirloom pendant. The more casual or creative your position, the more daring and trendy your jewelry options.

Jewelry Do's and Don'ts:

➤ Do stay away from dangling earrings, multiple rings, and noisy bracelets. Jewelry that moves too much or makes noise is distracting and will detract from any message you're trying to deliver.

➤ Do choose jewelry in proportion to your size. Teeny, tiny earrings, for example, will get lost on a large woman, while a jumbo brooch can overpower someone who's petite.

➤ Don't be afraid to mix silver and gold. They complement each other so well that some jewelry features both metals.

➤ Ditto fine and costume jewelry; gold-plated pieces often pair well with the real McCoy.

➤ Don't wear all-matching jewelry, for instance, X-shaped gold earrings, an X-shaped gold pin, and a necklace with an X-shaped gold pendant. So much coordination looks unsophisticated. Instead, buy one of the three items and wear it solo or paired with some other piece of gold jewelry.

➤ Do keep you ankle unadorned, even if you're wearing pantyhose. Ankle bracelets run counter to a professional look.

➤ Because accessories draw attention, keep you hands nicely manicured when wearing rings and bracelets.

Fashion Footnote

Fine jewelry is made from precious metals, like gold, sterling silver, and platinum, often in combination with precious or semiprecious stones. Fashion or costume jewelry is made of plated metals, as well as other materials, such as cubic zirconia, glass, plastic, and rhinestones.

Visual Impact

Eyeglasses can do more than correct poor vision; the well-chosen frame can create a serious, intelligent, even powerful look. Clark Kent, aka Superman, used the device to great effect—as have others in real life. "Getting glasses has definitely helped my image," notes one young woman who recently joined the workforce. "People take me more seriously because the glasses make me look older." If you think your image could benefit from such a boost, know that specs aren't just for the vision-impaired anymore; lots of people wear glasses solely to take advantage of their ability to suggest intelligence and authority.

Classically shaped frames in tortoiseshell, metal, or darker-colored plastic are usually smart choices for any business environment. Light colored frames suit those with light hair and eyes, and vice versa. When choosing wire rims, opt for gold, copper, or bronze frames if you're blonde or red-headed; silver, chrome, and black, if your hair is silver, gray, or dark. The more creative your role in an organization, the bolder, brighter, thicker, and more daring your frames can be. Go too edgy though (for example, solid black "geek" glasses or multihued, oversized octagonals), and you'll risk second glances.

In addition to helping you project a particular look, frame shapes can also flatter your face and balance your features. To use them to your best advantage, avoid repeating your face shape with an eyeglass frame. For example, while aviator-style glasses will emphasize a long face, round- or square-shaped frames with visually widen and shorten it. To add definition to a too-square face, consider an oval or angular cat's eye style; to counterbalance a more rounded face, choose rectangular styles. And though a frame should generally be about as wide as the widest part of the face, one that's a bit narrower or wider will broaden your face respectively.

To keep glasses from overpowering you or looking like you bought them in the children's department, match them to the size of your face (big or small) and the delicacy of your features (fine or full). Ideally, the top rim of your frames should line up with your eyebrows. If your glasses only partially cover your brows, you may end up looking as if you have two pairs of eyebrows.

Fashion Footnote

Women who are always putting on and taking off their glasses may want to consider keeping them where they're always close by—on an eyeglass chain. They're affordably priced and available in very elegant jewelry. But like clothing patterns, eyeglass chains work best when they don't compete with necklaces or scarves.

The Fashion Police

If you wear, or are thinking of being fitted with colored contact lenses, be sure they look natural. Some brands produce a very artificial effect that can be eerily distracting.

Put Your Best Foot Forward

While there's no limit to how many pairs of shoes a person can have, those who work should have at least two pairs of shoes to see them through the workweek. (Trying to get by with just one pair, even if you keep them well maintained, isn't a good idea; you'll get longer wear if you alternate shoes—that is, wait a day before you wear the same pair again.)

Women: Pump It Up

Most women who wear suits to work will need a pair of classic pumps in a neutral color that coordinates with their clothing. Black, navy, brown, or cordovan are good shoe hues. If the most casual you go is a pant suit, consider a sling-back-style shoe, or perhaps a two-toned spectator, as your second shoe choice.

How high a heel is too high? Perhaps less important than how high your heels are is how well you can walk in them (do you stride or wobble?) and what you wear them with (tailored separates or a tight blouse and short skirt?). Some women take advantage of higher heels to establish eye contact with male co-workers. (Even better, says one banker, is when men have to look up to meet her eyes!) But any confidence the heels bestow will be quickly undermined if you look as though you're going to topple over or the overall look is remotely suggestive. (Most women can easily maintain their equilibrium with 2-inch heels.)

Especially if you're on your feet all day, you'll want to know that the most comfortable heel height is anywhere from 1 to 1¹/₂ inches high; the wider the heel (even if it's higher), the more supportive it will be.

On casual days, flat loafers or oxfords (technically any shoe that ties) are handsome options—with or without chunkier heels. In general, the more substantial the shoe, the more professional it seems. Ballet style slippers or totally flat skimmers may be too lightweight. Another consideration: Not only do most women find that their legs are best flattered by a slight heel, they also find one to be more comfortable.

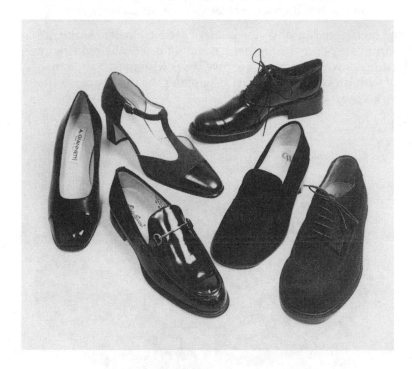

To climb the corporate ladder (clockwise from far left): Spectator pump, spectator T-strap, cap-toe oxford, suede wing tip, suede loafer, "bit" patent-leather loafer.

115

The Fashion Police

Low-cut shoes aren't any more acceptable than low-cut tops. For a shoe to look professional, it needs a high vamp, which means that the part of the shoe that covers the top of the foot should extend out at least a few inches from the base of your toes. Toe "cleavage" is a definite don't.

Men: Lace It Up

First and foremost, men in business suits need leather shoes that lace up. Oxford, as tie shoes are called, come in several styles: the traditional wing-tip, which has appliqued leather shaped like a bird's spread wings on the toe; the cap-toe oxford, that with an extra layer of plain or perforated leather across the toes; and the plain-toe oxford, which has no extra decoration. Each is dressiest in black, more casual in brown.

Less conservative but still dressy are slip-ons—the plain or tasseled loafer. At the opposite end of the spectrum are penny loafers, which should be considered strictly casual and are saved for dress down days. More creative types who need a shoe that can be worn equally well with dressy or softer suits may prefer the monkstrap, a slip-on shoe with a buckled strap across the instep.

What the well-heeled man is wearing (clockwise from front left): Tassel moccasin, cap-toe oxford (formal in black), wing tip, tassel loafer, cap-toe oxford (sportier in dark tan).

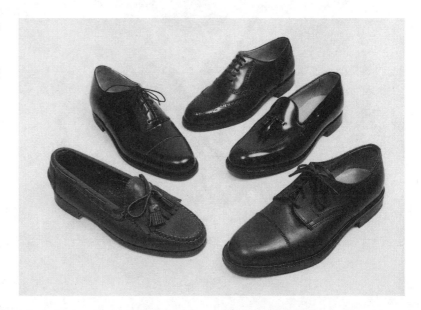

When a casual shoe is the order of the day (whether to pair with khakis or flannel trousers), loafers and oxfords—often in suede and with lug soles—work well. Depending on your office, a moccasin-style or modified deck shoe may also be appropriate.

Sock It to Me

There are four rules for sock wearers, be they male or female.

Fashion Footnote

Thin-soled shoes usually look more elegant than thick-soled shoes—for both men and women.

1. If you're going to match socks to something, make it your pants. But especially when wearing sportier garb, it's okay for socks to echo the colors of the clothing but not necessarily match (though that's okay too). There's nothing wrong, either, with patterned socks—so long as they're in keeping with the formality of your attire.

2. Very tailored or dressy clothing requires thin socks with a smooth or ribbed finish.

3. Socks should be high enough so that no calf or ankle skin gets bared when you sit down or cross your legs. For women, this requires knee-highs or trouser socks; men, over-the-calf socks.

4. Socks should match, be free of holes—and not be hanging on to respectability by a thread.

Fashion Footnote

Buy shoes in the late afternoon, when your feet are their largest and widest. Beware the salesperson who tells you that you have to break in a pair of shoes.

Ladies' Leg Work

Your choice of hosiery depends in large part on what type of shoe you're wearing. In conservative environments where classic pumps are de rigueur, the general rule of thumb is to wear sheer hosiery in a neutral tone—nude, black, or navy. Otherwise, you may prefer opaque hosiery, which both slims the leg and hides any unsightly veins or spots.

Wear sheer hosiery that's the same color as your shoes or lighter—but never white which flatters no one. One exception: when wearing a brightly colored garment, such as a red suit, match hosiery to shoes. Opaques work when slightly darker than you outfit.

Dollars & Sense

Three billion dollars a year is spent on women's hosiery.

Fashion Footnote

What's the difference between sheer and nude pantyhose? Sheer refers to the thickness of the yarn; nude refers to the color of the hose. Pantyhose come in a variety of nude tones, from beige to coffee—to accommodate a wide variety of skin tones. But not every nude-color hose is sheer, nor are all sheers nude; there are, for instance, nude opaques and black sheers.

Fashion Footnote

There are two ways to string a belt: Men are supposed to do it one way (inserting it from the left side), women the other (from the right).

What about wearing textured pantyhose? Though a quick way to perk up an outfit (without making a big financial commitment), even hose in traditional business patterns (like pinstripes, cables, and herringbones) may not be appropriate in conservative offices. Textures that probably won't get anyone a leg up: fishnets, bold crochets, metallics, free-floating dots, or florals.

The Belt Way

These days, when khakis are worn as frequently as pinstripes, it's nearly impossible to get by with just one belt. So have at least two on hand—one that coordinates with your dressiest apparel and one for casual wear. (The lighter the color, the less formal and dressy a belt looks.) The belt you'll wear on dress-down days can be made of suede, braided leather, canvas or twill; these types of belt usually runs a bit wider than their dressier brethren.

On days you're more formally outfitted, you'll need a belt in a fine-grade leather (preferably with a leather lining) that's related to the color of your shoes and is as dark as your clothes. If you want to increase the luxury quotient, choose an alligator belt or one with mock-croc embossing.

For working women who have more leeway with fashion, a gold chain mesh or animal-print belt looks classy and chic.

The most versatile buckles are understated, an especially wise option if your waist isn't an area to which you want attention drawing. They'll look less run-of-the-mill if they're not sporting initials. Gold, silver, brass, or matching leather are all work appropriate, with the latter being the most tailored. Matching your belt buckle to the rest of your jewelry, and accessories makes things easier.

Belts are sold according to waist measurements or in sizes small, medium, and large. One fits when it's long enough to reach the first loop but not the second, and if it feels comfortable when notched on the third hole. (Technically, these rules apply only to men's belts, but they make perfect sense for women, too.)

Brace Yourself

Suspenders, the American term for "braces," come in two styles: clip-ons and the kind that fasten to buttons via leather attachments. There's little doubt that the latter is the most elegant. But since all pants don't come readily equipped to accommodate button-on braces (though you or a tailor could sew on the buttons), clips may be your fate. No worries. More important is that your suspenders coordinate well with your tie and never be worn with a belt—it's an either/or situation. Avoid elaborate designs in wildy colorful suspenders, which are harder to match than a solid or subtly patterned pair, and can look clownish. (Remember Robin William as Mork?)

It's in the (Hand)bag

Ultimately, one good go-to-work handbag is all that a woman needs, and probably really wants, unless she doesn't mind transferring her belongings back and forth everyday. To really work, a purse should be big enough to hold all that you carry (but without bursting at the seams, bulging, or being out of sync with your size), coordinate with your clothes and other accessories (though not necessarily match your shoes), suit your style (can you sling it over your shoulder, or does it need to be carried by hand?), and stand up to daily use (think quality).

It should also be compatible with both your work and organizational style. If your clothes tend toward the traditional and tailored—gray flannel and navy suits—a structured, clean-lined, flap-top or bucket shoulder bag will go the distance. If sophisticated separates are your style, a drawstring tote, hobo style, or Kelly-type bag would be a good match. If your look is casual (khakis, sweaters, and tweedy jackets), a leather or nylon knapsack or saddle-style bag would work nicely. For the very organized, a bag outfitted with lots of compartments and pockets may be a must.

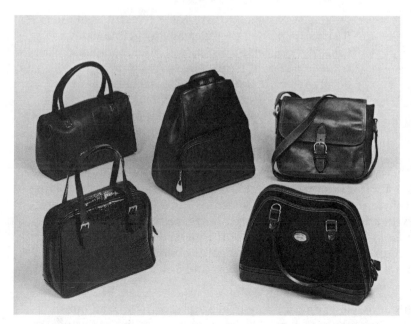

A handbag should fit your physique and hold the essentials. Some options (clockwise from top left): Double-handled bag, backpack, front-flap shoulder bag, Kelly-style bag, crocodile embossed handbag.

Structurally, look for firmly attached handles and straps (which look best if double-sided—that is, covered on both sides by the same material), reinforced stitching at stress points, well-secured zippers or snaps, and seams that are piped or bound. Top-grain leather—which is derived from the top layer of the hide and possesses its natural color—is the top-of-the-line grade, and handbags made of it are stronger and more durable than those made from split leather—the underneath layer of the hide, which is generally thicker and stiffer than top-grain leather.

The Fashion Police

How do you know whether your handbag "fits"? When selecting one, hold it upright across your stomach, with the top of it at your waist. The bag should fit between your hip bones and extend downward no farther than your crotch. If it extends beyond these perimeters, it's probably too large. A shoulder bag is too long if it hangs below your hip.

Fashion Footnote

The Kelly bag, named for Grace Kelly, was originally designed by the French fashion house, Hermès.

Getting Briefed

Originally designed for attorneys to carry legal briefs (hence the name), the briefcases available today to transport important papers and other paraphernalia come in a slew of handsome shapes and styles. So if you don't prefer the traditional rigid, rectangular cases (which can look clunky and cumbersome, especially when carried by women), your options include everything from knapsacks to satchels to soft-sided totes.

Materially speaking, leather is still the gold standard—pricey, but long lasting. If it doesn't fit into your budget, search out the best imitation leather you can find (some are remarkably real looking). In casual situations, canvas (especially with leather trim) and even tough nylon are acceptable substitutes. In any event, stay away from excessive hardware (in other words, anything that looks as though it would set off a metal detector or serve as a boat anchor) and choose a neutral color that coordinates well with your clothing and accessories. The most versatile briefcases have handles and a shoulder strap, which comes in very handy when your hands are full.

As for the sleek, aluminum-style briefcases, they're usually at odds with all but the trendiest of attire—plus they may make you look as though you're in the business of spying.

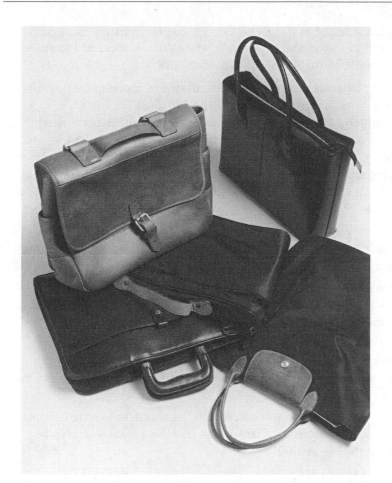

There are briefcases to suit all work styles.

The Fashion Police

Who needs a briefcase? You do, if you've been known to show up at important meetings carrying documents in a shopping bag or cardboard folder; your handbag is bursting at the seams with "homework"; everyone else carries one.

Accessories to the Crime

Though accessorizing is the key to elevating your look from just nice to downright natty, there is an art to getting it right. When chosen and worn just so, these finishing touches can transform any outfit; but if the execution is too far off, they can just as easily undermine it. So, what's the secret? It's no secret, really. All you need to succeed at accessorizing is an understanding of a few simple concepts:

➤ Though clothing can be accessorized to create a myriad of moods, the two components need to work together to create a specific look. For instance, a lugged-sole shoe can lend a sporty look to a pair of gray flannel pants just as easily as a mock-crocodile pump can dress them up. Sleek black accessories will give an urban edge to a basic beige suit, while a pretty floral-print scarf in cheerful colors will soften and feminize the look. It's when the message becomes mixed—i.e., you tote a structured black attaché case when wearing khakis and a polo shirt, or your old college knapsack with your business best—that an otherwise cohesive effect is ruined.

➤ Accessories shouldn't fight each other, particularly if they're worn nearby. One should be the most prominent, either in size or design.

➤ The bolder the design of an accessory, the more panache the wearer needs to carry it off—be it a bulky gold cuff or a tie with wide blocks of primary colors. Be sure you're up to the assignment.

➤ Accessories should not be overdone. (The old adage, less is more, definitely applies here.) Accessories used in moderation add style; too many create confusion. As a general rule, two pieces of jewelry near your face is plenty; this is a case of three's a crowd.

➤ Though you may not think of them as accessories, certain details—the color of a woman's nail polish, the buttons on a jacket, the bow on a shoe—need to be considered as part of the big picture.

The Least You Need to Know

➤ Accessories are an extension of your work wardrobe, and as such, they should be as carefully chosen as your clothing.

➤ Ties are the simplest and least expensive way for a man to accessorize and expand his wardrobe, and express his personality. Key considerations, due to their front-and-center positioning: high quality and precision typing.

➤ Scarves are to a women what ties are to a man: an easy way to add a dash of color or pattern to her outfit, and to completely change the look of the garments with which they're paired. They come in a myriad of sizes and can be worn many different ways.

➤ Jewelry worn on the job should never be distracting.

➤ For work, a classic timepiece—that is, one not outfitted with lots of doo-dads and gizmos—is most elegant.

➤ Leather accessories, including belts, handbags, shoes, and briefcases, should be in a color that coordinates well with your clothing. Though it's easier to match everything, it's not mandatory.

➤ Accessories need to be carefully integrated with clothing to create a cohesive look If an outfit somehow looks "off," rethink the accessories.

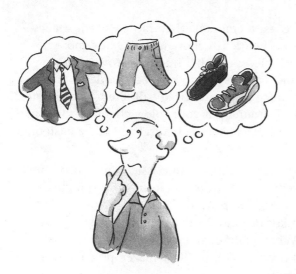

Chapter 10

So Many Options!

In This Chapter

➤ Wardrobe building do's and don'ts

➤ Three careers, three wardrobes

➤ Choosing complementary color

➤ Picking and incorporating pattern

So here you are, miles from where you began. You now know what in your closet is available for active duty, and the best options for filling in the gaps—in both clothing and accessories.

Still, there's more to learn: Exactly which pieces are musts for you—whether you're in accounting or advertising? How many suits (jackets, pants, shirts, skirts, and dresses) do you need in your wardrobe—to keep you from getting bored and your look from getting boring? Which neutral color should you build your wardrobe around—and how can you perk up the look without going overboard? All the answers are straight ahead, along with some savvy advice to keep you from taking missteps.

A Strategy for Success

The key to building a work wardrobe that you can count on is to invest in timeless pieces that mix and match to give you oodles of options. Some do's and don'ts:

➤ Do pick one or two neutral base colors around which to construct your wardrobe. Black, gray, navy, or camel are the best hues from which to choose. The logic:

Fashion Footnote

When just starting out in the work world, it's good to have at least a week's worth of clothing. From there, try budgeting for one or two items per month until you have another week's worth.

Neutrals are less memorable than more vibrant shades—and therefore, eminently more wearable and more mixable with pieces in other hues. Moreover, limiting clothing colors allows you to keep accessories to a minimum, since you won't need a different selection for each outfit. To round out your color scheme, choose two hues as accents, to offset the neutral and add a dash of excitement to the mix.

➤ Do opt for clothing cut in classic shapes. Anything too trendy (read oversized, form-fitted, pinched, boxy, flared, narrow, or otherwise exaggerated) won't last beyond the season and will date you—fast! What qualifies as a classic? Something that's stood the test of time, like a blazer, polo coat, or tailored trousers.

➤ Do keep clothing simple. The less details the better. That means no extraneous hardwear, unusual engineering, flounces, or appliques.

➤ Don't buy all solids. It may be a safer tact, but something patterned—even a simple stripe or small print not a bold-beyond-belief zebra motif—will add snap and help set you apart. Because they are so noticeable, you may want to reserve them for less-expensive items, like shirts and accessories—at least until you've got your core wardrobe needs taken care of.

➤ Don't buy fabrics that can't weather the seasons. Look for those, like tropical worsted wools and medium-weight cottons and silks, that work virtually year-round.

➤ Do buy the highest-quality garments that you can afford. Not only will they last longer, they'll look and feel better.

Determine Your Needs

The exact components of your work wardrobe will depend on your profession, your company's written or unwritten dress code, and your own preferences—including how frequently you can stand to repeat wardrobe. But to help get you on the right track, here are samples of three core wardrobes (in other words, the bare-bone essentials to get you through a workweek, including the occasional working weekend) for three distinctly different careers. One scenario should fit your work style.

In Corporate America

As an assistant VP in banking, you'll need a closetful of tailored suits at the ready—and for such a conservative profession, women's suits will likely need to be skirted. How many suits are required when you wear one everyday? Enough so that you don't have to repeat the outfit more than every three days. (Nothing holds up well to constant use, and wool suits especially, need to "air" a few days between wears.)

No matter what your profession, you should have enough shirts, blouses, or other tops to get you through the week. Men should stick with formal, fitted styles with spread or straight collars, in smoothly woven fabrics. Women can wear cotton or silk blouses and fine-gauge wool, silk, or cotton tops that layer nicely under a suit jacket. And since women also have the option of wearing dresses, a coat dress or sheath that matches a suit jacket provides a nice change of pace.

Fashion Footnote

If ties are an everyday thing at your place of business, aim to eventually have at least two per shirt.

If your otherwise sartorially uptight company has instituted a casual-day policy, you have several choices. At the dressiest end of the dress-down spectrum would be something along the lines of a navy or black blazer and gray flannel trousers, worn with a turtleneck or polo sweater. While this outfit would work for either sex, women could also pair a twinset or tunic with the trousers.

If khakis are kosher, males can wear a pair with a sport jacket (or that same blazer), an oxford-cloth shirt, and sweater; females may want to substitute a silk blouse for the rougher-textured shirt, and skip the sweater altogether.

The At-A-Glance Corporate and Conservative Man:

➤ Suits (at least three in all-season fabrics)

➤ Jackets (at least one sport coat, preferably a dark blazer)

➤ Pants (one dark wool flannel or gabardine and one pair khakis)

➤ Dress shirts (at least five, one for each workday, in various colors and patterns, preferably one with French cuffs)

➤ Casual shirts (one patterned, one white cotton both long-sleeved)

➤ Sweaters (one V-neck, one polo style)

➤ Accessories (classic wristwatch, cuff links, five ties in assorted patterns, pocket squares*, dressy and more casual leather belts, suspenders*, dressy leather lace-up shoes, casual leather or suede shoes, leather briefcase)

* Items are optional

The At-A-Glance Corporate and Conservative Woman:

➤ Suits (at least three, all with skirts; if pants are permitted, or you travel a lot, one suit should also have matching pants)

➤ Jackets (a dark blazer, one twinset)

➤ Pants (one dark wool flannel or gabardine and one pair khakis)

➤ Dress blouses/tops (at least one for each workday, including one in white cotton)

➤ Casual shirts (one long-sleeved with a convertible collar in silky fabric)

➤ Sweaters (one turtleneck)

➤ Dresses (a solid-colored sheath that matches a suit jacket)

➤ Accessories (classic wristwatch, tailored earrings, string of pearls, gold or silver necklace, cuff links, a square and an oblong scarf, leather belt, leather pumps, leather flats, leather handbag, leather brief-case or tote)

* Items are optional

Fashion Footnote

Make it your practice to buy shirts, ties, and any accessories at the same time you purchase a new suit. It's much easier to create winning combinations when you have all the pieces on hand.

On the Creative Side

As an account executive at a public-relations firm with an eclectic roster of clients, you have more latitude in how you dress, so softer, less structured suits and separates will form the basis of your wardrobe. The expected result: polished with personality and a higher trend quotient.

For client meetings, press events, and lunches with editors, a suit that works together with additional separates provides lots of mileage. For a Saturday afternoon book signing with an author/client, an unmatched jacket and pants with a mock-turtle sweater, fit the bill. When chained to your computer to churn out a press kit, khakis and a denim shirt over a white tee are comfortable, yet presentable; for a spur-of-the-moment meeting, just dress up the look by slipping on a dark blazer.

The At-A-Glance Creative Man:

➤ Suits (one in a solid color)

➤ Jackets (a dark blazer and a patterned sport coat that coordinates with suit trousers)

➤ Pants (one dark gabardine and one flannel, one pair khakis)

➤ Dress shirts (at least three white cotton)

➤ Casual shirts (one each: long-sleeved denim, polo, white tee)

➤ Sweaters (one mock turtleneck, one polo)

➤ Accessories (classic wristwatch, three ties, dressy and casual leather belts, dressy lace-up shoes, leather monkstrap shoes, leather backpack)

The At-A-Glance Creative Woman:

➤ Suits (one solid-color three piece: jacket, pant, and straight skirt)

➤ Jackets (one dark blazer and one patterned jacket that coordinates with suit pants and skirt)

➤ Skirts (one, perhaps with pleats, that works with two jackets)

➤ Pants (one each: dark gabardine, flannel, khakis)

➤ Dress blouses/tops (one each: silky blouse, white cotton shirt, silk shell)

➤ Casual shirts (one long-sleeved denim, one white tee)

➤ Sweaters (fine-gauge turtleneck and matching cardigan)

➤ Accessories (classic wristwatch; gold hoop earrings, gold studs; collar pin; one oblong, one square scarf; leather belt; leather pumps; suede flats; leather handbag; leather tote)

Did Someone Say Casual?

You wore a suit when interviewing for your position as a computer programmer, but haven't needed one since. Suits and other tailored clothing just isn't the company way; in fact, management has officially declared every day a casual day. You can wear jeans to your job (and others do without fail), but you usually prefer a more polished presentation. Because you also have to be prepared for the occasional out-of-the-office meeting with clients, at least one quasi-professional outfit is a must.

The At-A-Glance Casual Man:

➤ Jackets (one sport jacket or blazer that coordinates with two pairs of pants)

➤ Pants (one pair each: wool gabardine, wool flannel, corduroy, jeans, khakis)

➤ Shirts (one each: chambray, denim, corduroy, white cotton, patterned button-down, long- and short-sleeved cotton polo; two solid-color crewneck tees)

➤ Sweaters (one polo, one V- or crew-neck)

➤ Accessories (sporty wristwatch, two ties, leather belt, suede belt, leather oxfords, suede bucks, leather backpack)

The At-A-Glance Casual Woman:

➤ Jackets (one dark blazer or tweedy jacket and one twinset)

Fashion Footnote

If you have trouble coordinating individual items of clothing, take advantage of the fact that most stores and manufacturers sell clothing in small groupings in which everything mixes and matches. Usually displayed together or a single rack, it creates a very goof-proof system of shopping.

➤ Pants (two pairs of classic trousers, one pair of khakis, one pair each: jeans, knit pants)

➤ Skirts (one straight style, to coordinate with jackets)

➤ Shirts (two crisp cotton, one of them white; two silky; one denim or chambray; two solid-color crewneck tees)

➤ Sweaters (one turtleneck, one tunic-length pullover)

➤ Accessories (sporty wristwatch, one square and one oblong scarf, leather belt, suede belt, leather oxfords, suede loafers with slight heel, leather handbag, leather tote)

Cracking the Color Code

Now that your wardrobe needs are more or less sorted out, you have some colorful decisions to make—namely, which neutrals do you want to build your collection of clothing around, and which two or three colors would you like as accents, to provide some interest and contrast?

What should make it easier to decide is the fact that, despite what you may think or have heard about colors, there isn't one that you can't wear some variation of—provided it's the right temperature, intensity and clarity. If you're fond of gray, great; if brown is your favorite, that's fine, too. The tricky part is determining exactly which version of each color (charcoal gray or gunmetal gray? mocha or cafe au lait?) is the most complimentary to your own natural coloring.

Fashion Footnote

There's a whole language of color. "Value" refers to the lightness or darkness of color, or hue. "Clarity" refers to a color's brightness, which can be "muted" by adding gray. "Shades," "tints," and "tones" are all variations of colors that are formed by adding black, white, and gray, respectively, to a pure color. A "cool" hue has blue undertones, while a "warm" color has yellow.

The Fashion Police

Is red a neutral? If you define a neutral as a color that doesn't jump out at you and say hello, then red probably doesn't qualify—especially on men. (Who wouldn't notice Santa Claus?) That said, once a woman has put together a core wardrobe in say, navy or black, adding a red suit is perfectly acceptable—provided she's not in an industry that's very conservative.

Complimentary Colors: A Key

There are many systems for analyzing which colors work best for you. (Remember *Color Me Beautiful*?) In a nutshell, here's what they propose:

➤ A person's coloring is measured by how much yellow or blue is found in his or her skin, hair, and eyes. If you look best—that is, your skin seems clear, your eyes vibrant—in colors with blue undertones (for example, claret versus tomato red), you're considered "cool." If the opposite is true and yellow-based colors (brick versus rose) make you come alive, you're "warm." Be aware that there are warm and cool shades of every color, including neutrals. To determine which are most flattering, drape yourself in various shades of the same color and see how each affects your skin, hair, and eyes. (You may want to enlist your trusted friend or relative from Chapter 7, "Getting Started," to assist you in this color analysis.)

➤ Deeper, brighter shades look best on those with darker features (brown hair, brown eyes), while less-intense lighter or medium-toned shades are more flattering to those with softer or more muted coloring (blonde or graying hair, blue eyes).

➤ People with a lot of contrast between their skin, hair, and eyes (for example, they have steel-blue eyes, pale skin, and dark-brown hair) can carry off more dramatic color combinations—for instance, a black jacket and white shirt. People with low contrast (that is, light hair, skin, and eyes) require subtler, even monochromatic, color combi-nations—say, a beige-and-cream-checked

Fashion Footnote

Wearing a single color top to bottom creates a monochromatic look, one that's elegant and commanding—and that makes you appear slimmer and taller. To achieve the nicest effect, mix different textures.

jacket, beige trousers, and a cream-colored shirt. Those who fall somewhere in between (with, say, dark-brown hair, beigy skin, and hazel eyes) look best in combinations of light to medium (sky blue and charcoal gray) or medium to dark colors (dark brown and plum) or high or low contrast combinations with me-dium accent colors—navy and white with a deep periwinkle blue.

Accentuate the Positive

Every once in a while you've probably worn something to work that elicits the same response from everyone you see: "Wow, you look wonderful. That's a great color on you!" More likely than not, it was an accent color that provoked the positive reaction.

Accent colors are those that break up the monotony of neutrals and provide a bit of zip. Choosing one or two accents to complement a neutral color isn't that difficult.

131

Indeed, the beauty of neutrals is that they work with so many other colors. Gray, for instance, pairs well with red, blue, and yellow, as does beige, while black goes with virtually anything and everything. Still, that hardly means that effective accentuation is goof proof. Done poorly, the result is more comical than professional. What's the trick?

It's a matter of creating a pleasing contrast, an effect that's visually interesting, but never jarring. Sometimes it's as simple as choosing a soft or muted shade over one that's more vivid—say, dark forest green instead of acid green, butter yellow rather than citrus lemon, pumpkin instead of too-tangy orange. One easy way to successfully combine colors is to pair hues of like value—for example, heather gray and muted lavender, or chocolate brown and russet red.

To avoid looking like a kaleidoscope, you should also institute a no-compete clause when it comes to adding accents; too many different colors per outfit is distracting and can take away from your message.

Quote . . . Unquote

Blueneth doth express trueness.
...Ben Johnson

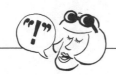

Fashion Footnote

What's not to like about dark colors? They minimize figure problems, hide dirt and stains, conceal less-than-perfect construction, and make cheap fabrics look more expensive.

Color Me ...

Authoritative? Approachable? Powerful? Serious? Colors can send messages about you and even influence the impressions you make on others. For instance, black and dark gray connote power and sophistication, dark blues telegraph strength, and bright, clear colors radiate energy.

The way you combine colors is equally powerful. The higher the contrast (say, wearing a white shirt under a navy suit), the more serious and authoritative you'll seem. To appear more receptive and approachable, go with lighter, muted shades (for example, pearl gray and soft yellow).

Color Key

Whether you're choosing a neutral or an accent, you'll always be flattered by colors that closely match those in your hair, skin, and eyes. If a color dulls, sallows, muddies, grays your skin, or makes you look remotely unhealthy, it's not one you should be wearing—at least not anywhere near your face.

Some other tips:

➤ Your best white should not be whiter or brighter than your teeth. On some people, the white that's most right is actually ivory or cream.

➤ Look closely at your eyes; even if they're technically blue, they'll usually contain an array of other colors—including yellow, green, gray, and brown. If a color is in your eye, it will be tremendously flattering when worn.

➤ If the dark ring that circles the colored part of your eye is navy, not black (as is true of many with brown eyes), navy will be particularly flattering on you.

➤ Your best red is the color on the inside of your lower lip.

Compounding Interest with Patterns

Though always correct, you can run the risk of looking dull, predictable, and devoid of creativity when repeatedly dressed in solid colors head to toe—even if one really catches your eye.

Enter pattern.

Patterns 101

Patterns can be woven or knit into fabric (usually a sign of higher quality) or printed on it after the fact. Either way, the world would be a more boring place if we didn't have them. Indeed, patterns provide much of the visual interest we get from clothing— be it a single splash on a tie, or the bolder mix of a shirt-and-jacket combination.

If the only pattern you're familiar with is the one that you see on your TV at three o'clock in the morning, this rundown on the various types—some of which are reserved for specific items like ties, whereas others work head to toe—will bring you up to speed.

Check Up

Checks is the term for all patterns made of crossing stripes. Some common checked patterns are:

➤ **Gingham**—A usually cotton fabric with stripes of equal width in two colors, one of which is generally white. The stripes intersect to create squares and a third color that's halfway between the two.

➤ **Houndstooth**—A pattern of even, broken checks, frequently in black and white.

➤ **Tattersall**—A pattern of narrow dark lines crossed to form squares on a white or contrasting colored ground.

Plaid Primer

A pattern is technically a plaid, which means blanket in Gaelic, when colored stripes or bars cross each other at right angles and form squares or blocks. Three classics are:

➤ **Glen plaid**—A pattern characterized by two checks of different sizes. It was named after Glen Urquhart, a valley in Invernessshire, Scotland.

➤ **Tartan**—A plaid of Scottish origin, formed when the threads that run lengthwise are arranged in precisely the same pattern as those that run widthwise, thus producing a balanced design. Think kilt, and you'll get the idea.

➤ **Windowpane**—Widely spaced stripes that resemble a multi-paned window.

See a pattern developing? From top: floral, paisley, herringbone, pinstripe, pencil stripe, chalk stripe, tartan, Glen plaid, polka dot, gingham, houndstooth, foulard, regimental stripe, tattersall, windowpane.

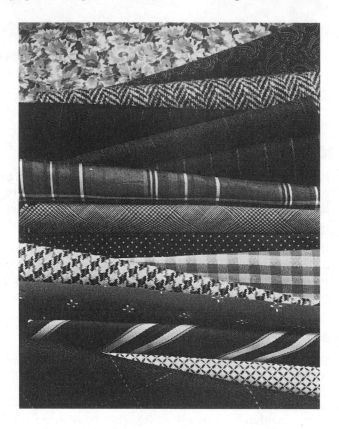

Learning Your Stripes

A design consisting of bands or straight lines against a plain background, there are many types of stripes:

➤ **Chalk stripe**—White stripes of varying widths that resemble chalk lines.

➤ **Pencil stripe**—A dark, narrow stripe on a lighter background.

➤ **Pinstripes**—Very narrow lines (the width of a straight pin) created by a succession of dots.

➤ **Regimental stripe**—Diagonal stripes, so called because they were worn by English regiments in certain indentifying colors.

Pattern Potpourri

Some other patterns that don't fit precisely into one of the other three categories are also very popular. They include:

➤ **Floral**—Any pattern in which flowers predominate.

➤ **Foulard**—A small geometrical design on a plain background.

➤ **Herringbone**—A pattern with a sideways zigzag or chevron effect.

➤ **Paisley**—A curvy pattern of amoeba-like shapes that derives from the shape of the date palm tree.

➤ **Polka dots**—Round spots of any size; the most common version is white dots on a colored background.

Fashion Footnote

The most popular pattern of business is probably pinstripes, which may have been inspired by the lines in accounting ledgers.

Picking Patterns

Creating the right effect with patterns requires equal parts daring and control, along with the good judgement to recognize an effort gone awry. The goal: To turn up the creative volume just enough to create some sartorial excitement—and to set you apart from the flair impaired. The risk: Going overboard and blasting your co-workers out of their chairs. Such disastrous results can be avoided by taking note of a few guidelines:

➤ Especially if you're in a conservative field or have a limited wardrobe, subtle patterns are more versatile and less obvious. For instance, a herringbone or chalk stripe is less memorable than an oversized floral or geometric design (or the tea-cup design recently spotted on a blouse), which—after being worn a few times—will certainly lose its novelty. No matter what your line of work, splashy prints, wide colorful stripes, and loud plaids should generally be avoided like the plague.

➤ A small dose of a pattern can go a long way, especially if it's strong or busy. That's why a sports jacket in herringbone works and a similarly patterned suit often doesn't. Avoid patterns that overwhelm or that appear to be wearing you.

➤ Generally, smaller, darker patterns are dressier and more conservative; louder, brighter, and bigger patterns are best suited to casual attire.

Fashion Footnote

When nothing but solids will do, an interesting combination of textures (like the ribs woven into a corduroy jacket juxtaposed with the sleekness of a silk shirt) can replace a pattern.

135

➤ Never assume that just because a pattern has a multitude of colors in it that you can pair it with a garment in any of those colors. Oftentimes, a pattern really works with only one color.

➤ Patterns in contrasting colors, like white and black, can be fatiguing to the eye—especially when the pattern is large.

➤ Coordinate your patterns to your personality and physical stature: A slim, shy, retiring type looks conspicuous in larger, louder patterns and vice versa.

Combining Patterns

If your idea of wearing pattern is to add a stripe tie to a solid suit and shirt, join the club. There are lots of people coordinated enough to juggle three assignments at once who aren't adroit at combining two patterns—be it stripes and dots or stripes and stripes. But learning how to merge and acquire patterns in a business wardrobe may signal that you can think outside the box. These guidelines should prevent you from creating any pulsating effects when combining patterns.

➤ Patterns should be in the same color family as your solid pieces.

➤ With stripes, success comes from varying the widths, as well as having a color in common. For instance, if your shirt has a thin stripe, pair it with a boldly striped tie.

➤ Scale is also key; when mixing two patterns, one should be larger than the other.

➤ Unless you're supremely confident in your ability, stick with two patterns per outfit. Though three patterns can certainly be successfully combined, it can be risky business. Work on developing your eye before going public.

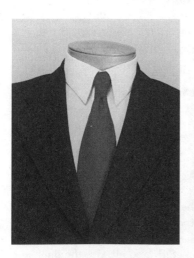 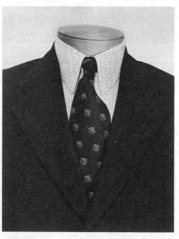 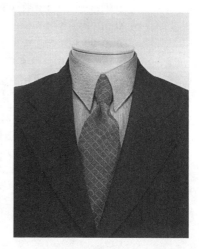

A dark suit is always correct with a white shirt and solid tie, but pairing one with patterned shirts and ties makes it more interesting.

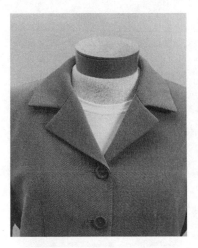 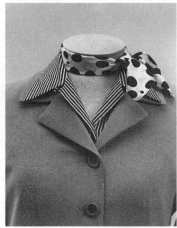 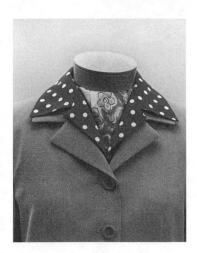

Stripes, polka dots, and florals take a solid suit from safe to snappy.

The Least You Need to Know

➤ When building a wardrobe, it's best to buy classically styled core pieces in neutral colors (like black, brown, navy, gray, camel, or beige) and seasonless fabrics.

➤ Precisely which pieces you'll need in your work wardrobe will depend on what you do, how casual your work environment is, and your personal preferences.

➤ There are no right or wrong choices; everyone can wear practically any color, provided it complements his or her natural pigmentation.

➤ Accent colors, which provide contrast to a neutral outfit, can be bright or muted. Used to best effect, they don't overwhelm the wearer or the outfit.

➤ Patterns add visual interest to an outfit and come in a wide variety. To successfully mix patterns, stay in the same color family and keep one of the patterns more dominant than the others.

Chapter 11

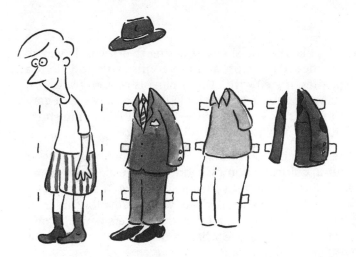

Milking Your Wardrobe for All It's Worth

In This Chapter

➤ A suit: more than the sum of its parts

➤ Exercising options

➤ Don't discriminate

Having spent my formative fashion years wearing a school uniform, I can remember how difficult it was to make the same old thing look anything but. Every morning, it was the same mission: Turn the plaid skirt and white blouse into an outfit that looked different—at least from how it looked the day before.

Oddly enough, things haven't changed much today. Now, as then, the goal is to make the most of some basic pieces, to greatly multiply their wearability. What does it take to maximize the often enormous untapped potential of what's already hanging in your closet? Two things that don't cost a dime, yet provide high-yield dividends: a fresh perspective and a healthy dose of creativity. In case you're feeling fresh out, some inspiration for both is included in this chapter.

Frankly, though, these concepts are hard to explain in words alone, which is why the second half of this chapter—four full pages—is filled with idea-packed photographs. Because, while how-tos on getting the most mileage from your work wardrobe are helpful, a picture is worth thousand words—and will get your creative juices flowing that much faster.

Break Up a Pair

A lot of people mistakenly treat suits like they do shoes, thinking that the only way to wear the two pieces is together. But these days, more and more suits can stand alone as separates, mixed with other elements of your wardrobe to take on a entirely new look: Pair the jacket with gray flannels, khakis, or jeans; the pants with a denim shirt, knit polo, or white button-down shirt.

The best candidates for successful separation are suits in neutral colors, seasonless fabrics, and relaxed silhouettes. But don't limit yourself. There aren't any rules for what will work. The only way you'll know for sure is to give it a whirl: Try on all your suit jackets with all your pants or skirts and see what works. Then do the reverse with your suit bottoms.

I once went through this exercise when I was beginning a new job at the same company and wanted to freshen up my look. Frankly, because I had so few clothes to begin with, I couldn't imagine that I'd discover a great outfit hidden away in my closet. But in a moment of sartorial clarity, I realized that the plain wool skirt that I had previously worn only with a dressy jacket would work perfectly without its matching mate. The next day, I paired that skirt with a blouse and cardigan and—presto!—a new outfit was born.

Fashion Footnote

One tip for successfully re-pairing a suit jacket or pant: Colors and textures needn't match exactly, but should coordinate or harmonize—try a navy jacket with camel trousers or a plush, heathered flannel with a heavy tweed.

Consider All Possibilities

As creatures of habit, it's easy to fall into the trap of regarding your wardrobe as a series of outfits. Each time you wear a certain pair of pants, you reach for the same shirt, sweater, and/or jacket—even though there are other options in your closet. And why not? It's so easy, you could do it in your sleep (and sometimes you may actually be half-asleep when you do!).

There is no doubt that people need tried-and-true outfits, the ones that they can reach for when they've overslept or have too much on their minds to get creative with their clothing. But as a rule, the if-it's-Monday-it-must-be-the-brown-pants-with-the-cream-shirt approach to dressing defeats the purpose of building a working wardrobe—one that, in this case, would also contain a blue shirt to go with the brown pants. It's also a surefire way to bore you, and possibly everyone in your department, to tears.

Fashion Footnote

If a refashioned outfit doesn't seem to be working, try pulling it together with accessories. The right belt or tie can often unify some otherwise incompatible elements.

How do you stop pigeonholing your clothes and start taking advantage of their versatility? Again, it's a matter of spending some time trying on your clothes without any preconceived notions about what goes with what; this is the time to look at things in a new light and reassess their potential. Ignore the little voice in your head that tells you that the plaid jacket couldn't possibly work with the checked pants. Maybe it can't. But at the very least, the process of trying to put the two together may spark another idea for a working combination.

Attitude Readjustment

Are you guilty of stereotyping, the very common and extremely limiting tendency toward only pairing like with like, for instance, a silk blouse with something equally dressy (instead of using it to add polish to a pair of khakis or corduroys) or jeans exclusively with sporty counterparts (when a velvet blouse would raise them to a new level of elegance)? If so, you're likely cutting your outfit options in half, plus, missing out on opportunities to go beyond the expected. Often times, it's the juxtapositioning of fabrics and silhouettes that makes outfits look more interesting and less ordinary.

There's no better time than now to knock down the barriers in your closet. As business attire moves toward the casual, merging the informal (a fitted T-shirt and khakis) with the traditionally formal (a navy jacket) is the key toward wardrobe expansion without additional expense.

Fashion Footnote

You can add new life to a garment by wearing it differently. Push up the sleeves of a jacket or a shirt, or flip up the lapels. Look at shirts with an eye for layering them with other shirts or sweaters. Sweaters can be tucked in or belted, or draped over the shoulder, for a new look.

Exercise in Utility

Putting these principles of wardrobe expansion into practice will be far easier if you have some inspiration, and that's what the next pages are about. Each page tackles a different assignment, but the goal is the same: to get the most out of your work clothes.

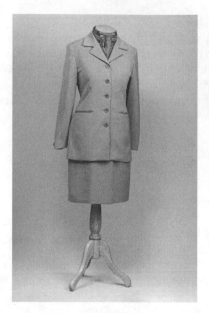

One suit, four looks. Simply sophisticated with a silk scarf. (Suit courtesy of JCPenney.)

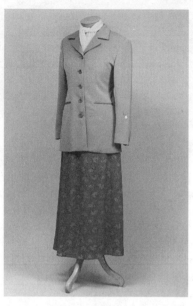

A pretty, polished look. (Skirt courtesy of Liz Claiborne Collection.)

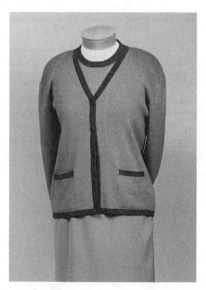

A twinset stands in for the jacket. (Twinset courtesy of JCPenney.)

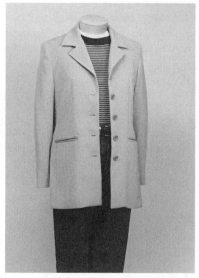

The jacket dresses up jeans and a tee. (Jeans courtesy of Eddie Bauer.)

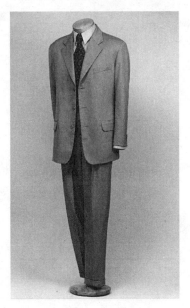

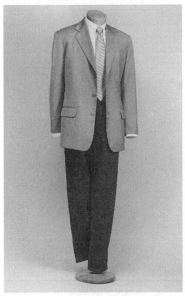

How versatile can one suit be? The jacket and trousers combined for maximum impact and formality. (Suit courtesy of Claiborne.)

Jeans look most professional when worn with a jacket and tie. (Jeans courtesy of Eddie Bauer, tie courtesy of Lands' End.)

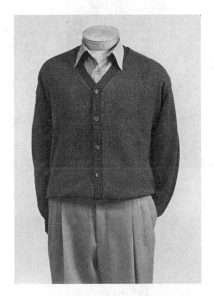

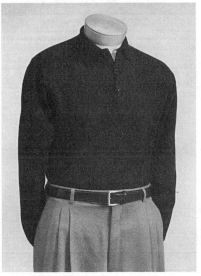

A shirt and cardigan relax the trousers ...

... which look sleek paired with a dark polo sweater.

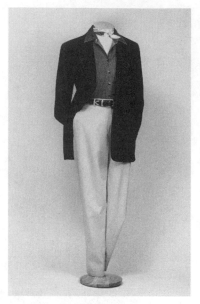

The many faces of khakis. Looking sharp with a denim shirt and navy blazer ...

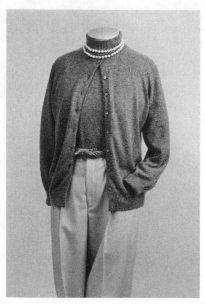

... and elegant teamed with a twinset and pearls.

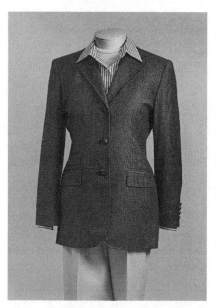

Classy and cultured ...

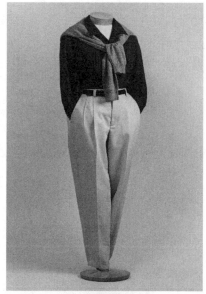

... sporty, yet smart.

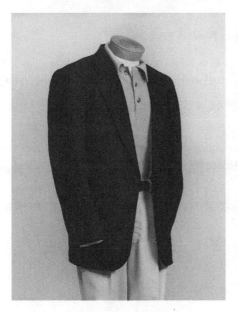

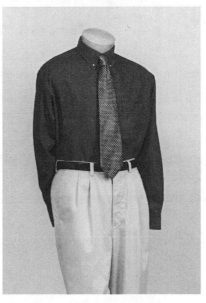

Don't pigeonhole these pants. Khakis work with a jacket (Blazer courtesy of Eddie Bauer.) ...

... and a tie. (Tie Lands' End, shirt courtesy of Eddie Bauer.)

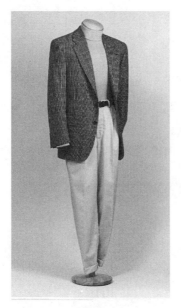

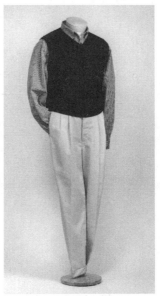

When a suit's too stuffy (Turtleneck courtesy of Lands' End.)...

... and no jacket's required.

The Least You Need to Know

➤ There's no rule that says suit pieces always have to be worn together. To get the most mileage, disassemble them and try pairing each part with other separates.

➤ Thinking of your wardrobe as a series of outfits is very limiting. Mix and match pieces to expand your options.

➤ Your wardrobe will live up to its maximum potential if you're open-minded about how you wear your clothes. Relegating certain garments to specific uses drastically reduces their value.

Part 4
Special Performances

Despite the day-in, day-out importance of how you dress, on certain occasions the matter requires some rethinking or even gets elevated to a new plane. Take the job interview. Because more is riding on how you're dressed when meeting a potential employer than at any other time, Chapter 12, "The Job Interview," is a must-read for job seekers.

If you find yourself being invited (or summoned!) to meetings, receptions, and industry galas, you'll find Chapter 13, "Out of the Office, but Still on the Job," chock-full of helpful advice. Check it out, too, for suggestions on salvaging your dignity at the company picnic.

When you feel the need for the information in Chapter 14, "When All Eyes Are on You," you'll know you've reached a certain level in your career. That's because Chapter 14 deals with presenting a professional public persona, specifically when you're speaking in front of a group; appearing on a TV show; or being photographed for a newspaper, magazine, or newsletter. All of these situations present special wardrobe challenges. But don't worry; when opportunity comes knocking, you'll be ready!

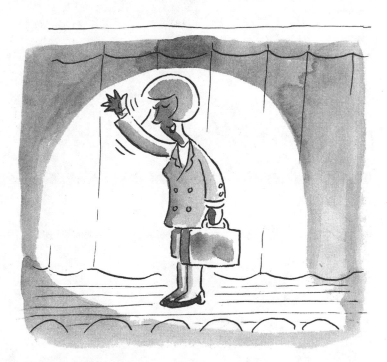

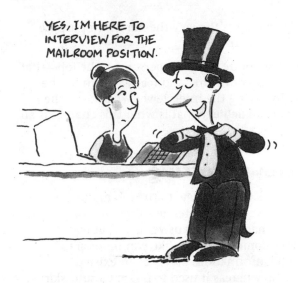

YES, I'M HERE TO INTERVIEW FOR THE MAILROOM POSITION.

Chapter 12

The Job Interview

In This Chapter

➤ It's show time!

➤ Be safe, not sorry

➤ No detail too small

➤ The second interview

You just got the call: "We've reviewed your résumé and would like to meet with you about the sales position." Hooray! You've made it over the first hurdle. Up next, the job interview. Or, as many refer to it, the *dreaded* job interview.

As it turns out, job seekers are right to be anxious about interviews—especially the first few seconds of one. As interviewers readily acknowledge, they draw conclusions based on how you look just an instant or two after you walk through the door. From then on, everything you do is used to strengthen that initial impression—whether it's deserved or not. Be dressed in a sophisticated manner and some small blunder, say, tripping on the carpet, gets attributed to your enthusiasm and eagerness. Come outfitted in a rumpled, outdated outfit, however, and the same stumble becomes further confirmation of just how wrong you are for the job. "Right or wrong, you tend to cut people some slack if they come in dressed appropriately," admits one manager.

With so much riding on it, a job interview is certainly the occasion to pull out all the stops, sartorially speaking, to send the right message. "When meeting someone for the first time, what you wear is a statement of what you want them to know about you," notes one director of human resources. "People dress the way they dress on purpose, and that's the message the interviewer is faced with."

What you want your appearance to say is that you're the right person for the job—that you're sharp, competent, reliable, serious about your work, and ready to handle the additional responsibility. How to do that? By giving the interviewer what he or she wants to see: your best impression. How you can achieve that is what this chapter is all about.

The Inside Track on Interview Dressing

If you haven't interviewed for a job in a few years or are new to the job market, you're probably wondering whether the rules that have guided interview dressing for the last 20 years have changed. The answer is yes, at least for certain fields—some of which, like computer graphics and electronic information, barely even existed two decades ago. So whereas it used to be that a suit (skirted for women) in dark blue or gray was de rigueur at interviews, today there is more flexibility from industry to industry as to what attire meets the standard of acceptability.

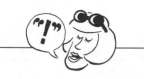

Quote . . . Unquote

When you go to an interview, that's the time! ...Harris Shephard, owner of Harris Shephard Public Relations

What hasn't changed is your overriding goal—to present a polished, professional appearance. Even if you can dress informally once hired, raising the bar for the interview shows a certain amount of respect—which will not go unnoticed. "I want to see some effort. If someone is applying for a job and they don't give me their best the first time in the door, they're certainly not going to do it for the rest of their employment," says one company president.

Indeed, a prospective employee who doesn't make the effort is doing himself or herself a real disservice. Such was the case when a woman dressed in shorts and a chambray shirt came before a board charged with hiring a park and recreation director in a rural area of the Northeast. "If this woman was a professional, she would have know that, while she never would have been required to dress that way on the job, a higher standard should be set for an interview," says one on the board members.

Must You Suit Up?

Posed with the question "What should someone wear to a job interview?" those in a position of hiring all said virtually the same thing: Wear what's appropriate for the industry—and the position—for which you are interviewing. Does that always require that you wear a suit? Not necessarily. Though in most situations, playing it safe with a suit is strongly encouraged, in some instances, doing so may be a sign of ignorance—of not having done your research and, as a result, not having a sense of what the corporate environment is like.

Where a matched suit may not be a necessity is in an industry that's celebrated for its casualness. "I do a lot of searches for small Internet companies in Silicon Valley. They are very casual, extremely so. As a result, because it wouldn't fit in with the tone of the company, I don't recommend that my clients wear a suit. Still, since you don't know the individual with whom you're interviewing, you have to be cautious," advises a recruiter at an executive search firm.

Suitable Attire

Indeed, if ever there was a buzzword to guide you in your quest to make a great impression at a job interview, it's caution. As acceptable as it is to allow some of your personality to come across in how you dress, it's far more important to wear something that says interview. Whatever your industry, it's important to understand the parameters within which you should dress.

In some instances, particularly ultraconservative areas like the law and finance, there's little doubt that a traditionally tailored suit—typically, a dark, neutral-colored, single-breasted jacket with matching skirt or pants—is the outfit of choice. To show you mean business, team it with a crisp, long-sleeved, white shirt (or a more fluid silk blouse or shell for women), a small-patterned tie (or elegant necklace or pearls for women), and dark, tie shoes (or closed-toe pumps for you-know-who).

Fashion Footnote

Dark colors suggest authority, and dark blue conveys the greatest degree of authority. What about black? It may be considered too dark and somber for a job interview. Red? Too bold.

In more creative fields such as marketing, advertising, and graphic design, dressing too conservatively could actually be detrimental to your campaign. For instance, in my field, the editorial, or "creative," arm of publishing, the aforementioned suit would look too stodgy. A better option here would be an ensemble in a businesslike fabric, but with some untraditional touches. Think of a suit that reflects the wearer's personality and creativity, albeit quietly, and you get the picture.

Dark blue or gray isn't a must, though a neutral tone certainly looks more serious. A subtle pattern is acceptable, as is pairing a solid suit with an elegantly patterned shirt and tie. Just save anything too bold for another occasion where the stakes aren't as high and you're certain not to offend anyone's sensibilities. "Fashion may be universal, but taste is individual. You don't want to take any chances by dressing too eclectically or outlandishly," notes one sales manager.

At an ultracasual firm (we're talking some place like Microsoft or Nike, where jeans and sneakers aren't out of place and are often the norm), or in a field like teaching where you want to be seen as intelligent but very approachable, a jacket and pants or skirt that coordinates, but doesn't necessarily match, shows due deference and is in keeping with the relaxed environment.

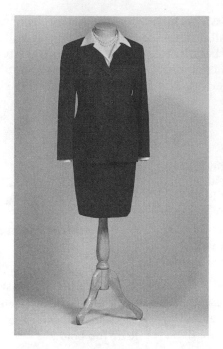 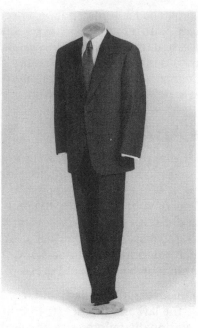

Making the right impression at a conservative company (Woman's suit courtesy of Talbot's; man's suit courtesy of Lands' End.) ...

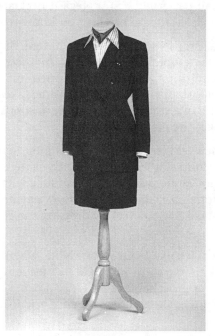 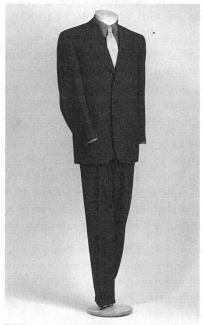

... in a creative field (Woman's suit courtesy of JCPenney; man's suit courtesy of JCPenney.)

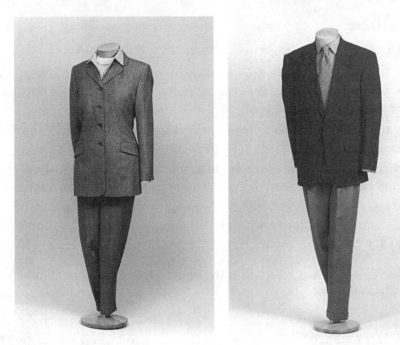

... where the dress code is casual. (Woman's and man's clothing courtesy of AKA Eddie Bauer.)

No Matter What

Whatever position you're interviewing for, no matter what industry it's in, there's one unbreakable rule: Always dress for the position you're seeking, not the one you already have. "It's remarkable how looking the part can make up for not actually being qualified to do it," said an administrator.

If you're not sure how an employee in the position you're interviewing for dresses, do some investigating. Ask your friends in the industry, or a trusted colleague employed at the company. If you're working with a recruiter, certainly ask and carefully consider his or her advice.

The Fashion Police

Dresses, especially those worn with a matching jacket, are appropriate for interviews. "That they so closely approximate a suit makes them perfectly acceptable," notes one human resources manager.

When in Doubt

With interviewing comes uncertainty. Consider these four quandaries:

1. You're scheduled to interview on a Friday, the day set aside by many otherwise conservative companies for dressing down. To avoid looking out of place, should you loosen things up a bit, too?

2. You're not certain whether a particular firm prefers skirts for female applicants. You favor pants. Should you wear a pair?

3. You've sported an eyebrow earring since your college days, when you and your fraternity brothers got pierced on a dare. Can you wear it to an interview?

4. You're just out of college, have little disposable income, and are considering wearing your best button-down shirt, sweater, tie, and khakis to an interview. Should you risk it?

The answer to each of these questions is the same—a resounding no! But let's address them in detail one by one.

Answer #1.

"Unless you're specifically told to dress casually, do so and you'll risk starting things off on the wrong foot," says a human resources manager, who doubts that an applicant would ever be instructed to dress down. "It's not encouraged because it's just not the same presentation." Worried that you'll feel uncomfortable being the sole suit in a sea of denim? Rest assured: You may be overdressed for their environment on that particular day, but you'll be appropriately dressed for an interview.

The Fashion Police

Save anything with polka dots for after you land the job. Even the most demure dots might not look serious enough at an interview.

Answer #2.

If you're unsure whether pants will fall outside the boundaries of acceptable dress at an interview, by all means, wear a skirt. It's not unusual for companies that normally permit pants to find them objectionable at an interview. One executive at a conservative company recalled a situation in which a woman who was otherwise qualified for a position didn't get the nod because she came to the interview in a pants suit. "It struck me and my associates as wrong that she was dressed the way she was. It would be fine attire around the office—we don't wear suits here everyday. But I would never show up for an interview in pants."

Answer #3.

Actually, you could wear the earring, but chances are that—like most bold cultural statements—it could turn off the interviewer. Whether you could wear it if you did get the job is another issue, and one that you eventually might have to tackle.

Answer #4.

You might get away with it—"I recently hired a fellow who didn't wear a jacket to the interview. The way I looked at it was that he was a young kid, and for the position he was interviewing, looked fine," reports a manager in a small office—but why chance it? You'll risk less if you spring for a jacket and dress pants. Don't worry about buying the most expensive clothing; choose garments in neutral colors that look smart and fit you well, and you'll rate higher on the good-impression meter.

I speak from experience here. For my first interview out of college (at *McCall's* magazine), I put a big dent in my Macy's credit card by buying a blue suit, pumps, and two blouses in completely different styles that would, I hoped, make the suit—the only one I owned—look as different as possible. I wore this suit to two interviews at *McCall's* and ultimately got the job. Shortly thereafter, my boss mentioned in passing that my effort to look professional had counted for a lot. Not only had she correctly surmised that each garment I had worn had been purchased especially for the interviews, she had factored it into her decision to hire me!

The Fashion Police

Height commands authority, which can be used to great advantage in an interview. Shorter women who are comfortable wearing a slightly higher heel ($2^1/_2$ inches, tops) should do so; wearing lifts is a personal decision for the vertically challenged male. No matter what your height, concentrate on carrying yourself well. Don't slouch, stoop, or walk with your head down. Stand tall, walk proud!

The Devil Is in the Details

If ever there was a time for shoes to be shined, hair to be trimmed, and clothes to be neatly pressed, it's the job interview. Not that anyone needs to feel any more pressure

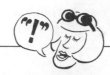

Quote . . . Unquote

There are some positions for which I've had companies say, "It really doesn't matter how the person dresses for the interview." Now, you can say that, but if two people walk in with the same set of credentials, the better-dressed person will probably get the nod. ...Jackie Riley of Lynne Palmer Associates, an executive search firm

when preparing for an audience with a prospective employer, but it's important to know that oftentimes it's the little things an interviewer notices that undermine your chances for landing the spot you covet.

Case in point, related by a human resources manager: "I recently brought in a man to interview for vice president of marketing, a position that's all about packaging. He pulls out this eyeglass case that looks like it's been through the war. One of the other employees who had also interviewed this man asked me later if I had seen the eyeglass case—it made that much of an impression. No doubt, the applicant thought, it's just an eyeglass case. But people will notice—and never forget—if something is particularly shoddy or completely out of style, or if someone looks disheveled or unkempt."

Interview Don'ts

What are the most common fashion slip-ups seen in interviews? Here, the top 10:

1. **Uncomfortable clothing**—Let's face it, there are very few people who are professional interviewers, and it can be a tense situation, so you want to be as comfortable as possible (remember, comfort breeds confidence). That means that whether it's borrowed or brand new, avoid wearing anything to an interview that you've never worn before. You need a trial run to determine whether a garment pulls funny when you lean forward, or is too low cut, gapes in the wrong places when you extend your arm—so you can choose something less bothersome to wear if it does.

2. **Unpolished shoes**—Many people subscribe to the theory that you can be summed up by the state of your shoes. Just in case your interviewer does, too, don't wear a pair that's in a sorry state. Check for worn heels and scuffs. To put your best foot forward at an interview, men should wear tie shoes, women, closed-toe shoes with moderate heels.

3. **Hosiery with snags, runs, or holes**—It may be better than no hosiery at all (a definite don't), but hardly, so check carefully before heading out. In case Murphy's Law gets the better of them, women should always carry a spare pair of pantyhose in their handbags, briefcases or glove compartments.

4. **Heavy cologne or perfume**—You don't want to overwhelm or nauseate the interviewer.

5. **Electric colors**—Sure, everyone will see you coming, but that's not exactly your goal. To be memorable for the right reasons, wear bright (not brilliant) colors strategically, as accents.

6. **Excessive or distracting accessories**—Remember that less is always more. Restrict yourself to a few tasteful adornments.

7. **Overdone hair or unnatural makeup**—Maintain a light touch with the mousse and mascara. And while we're on the subject, make sure nothing about your hair is distracting. "I interviewed a woman who had a long strip of hair dangling over her eye. I just wanted to reach over and brush it off. I was thinking that she had to have seen it when she looked at me, but she sat through the whole interview and never moved it," relates an administrator.

8. **Too-dressy clothes**—Wearing cocktail suits, blouses with lace collars, or anything just this side of formal will make you look as though you're attending a wedding later in the day—a situation one woman encountered when interviewing a prospective employee. "She came in wearing a black cocktail dress because she was going out immediately afterward. Talk about taking liberties."

9. **Overflowing bags or briefcases**—"I want someone who looks organized, not someone carrying a briefcase that's bulging at the seams or that has papers hanging out," notes an executive director of a foundation. Pare down to the essentials and, so you don't look like you just schlepped cross-country, try to carry it all in one bag—preferably a briefcase, which conveys authority.

10. **Neglected nails**—If you're not good with your hands, this might be a good time to splurge on a manicure.

Dollars & Sense

Should you buy something totally different from your usual work garb to interview at a company that's more or less conservative than your current employer? Only if nothing in your wardrobe is suitable—that is, makes you feel terrific. Even then, try to limit any investment; maybe a new tie or blouse would suffice, at least until you're asked back for the second interview.

Countdown to the Interview

The morning of the interview is not the time to sort through your wardrobe to find the perfect something to wear. Here's a better plan to look like you're the person for the job:

➤ **The day you line up the interview**—Assess your clothing options and determine the possibilities. (Don't forget accessories.) Repair loose hems, replace missing buttons, and determine what needs to go to the cleaners. Take inventory on your stock of pantyhose and socks. If necessary, schedule an appointment for a haircut or color touch-up at least a few days before the interview—just in case you experience any tress distress that requires repairs.

➤ **The next day**—Hit the stores for items you need to complete your outfit.

➤ **That night**—Have a dress rehearsal. To be sure nothing is out of synch, take this test: Close your eyes for five seconds and then open them and look at your reflection in a mirror. The goal: Nothing should jump out at you; if something does (for example, a bulging shoulder pad, a too-loud tie, patterned hosiery), remove or change it.

➤ **The evening before**—Shine your shoes; press and lay out your clothes.

➤ **The morning of**—Shower, so you're at your freshest.

➤ **Ten minutes before**—What you do or don't do in these pre-interview moments could help you win the job, or—as the following three real-life cases illustrate— potentially cause you to lose it. In the first, a man travelling by plane to an interview sits next to a woman eating chicken wings. During the interview, the interviewer informs him that he has a piece of chicken on his lapel. In the second, a female candidate shows up in a new suit, something that was apparent to the interviewer since there was still a sales tag hanging from underneath her arm. In the third, a man arrives for his interview a few minutes early and proceeds to wet shave in the restroom. Unfortunately for him, the president of the firm happens upon him and relays the tale to the manager of human resources. The moral of these stories? Do use the few minutes you have prior to the interview to visit the restroom, where you can touch up your hair and makeup, and check for dandruff flakes, lint, and stray threads (and tags!). Don't expect to perform an overhaul on yourself in there.

Weathering the Interview

You can't expect the weather to cooperate when you have an interview scheduled. In fact it's best to be prepared for the worst. "Employers expect you to be able to dress for the weather, and canceling because of the weather could be held against you," notes a human resources director. If rain or snow does come to pass, stash your boots and umbrella in a tote bag that you can leave in the coat closet or with the receptionist.

What to do when the unthinkable happens, and you fall victim to a splash-and-dash motorist? Unless it's an out-and-out disaster, don't cancel. Instead, remove as much of the much as possible in the restroom, and then casually make mention of the incident to the interview *before* he or she has the chance to bring it up. Maintain you sense of humor ("I don't usually like to interview in muddy pants, but this inconsiderate driver had other ideas"), and your candor and composure will be duly noted.

The Spur-of-the-Moment Interview

It's an unlikely scenario, but it's possible that you'll get a last-minute call to come in and interview on a day when you're casually dressed. "We've had calls for candidates to go on interviews when we've caught them off guard in the office and they're wearing jeans," says one recruiter.

If you won't have enough time to go home and change your clothes, explain that although you'd be happy to come in (if, in fact, you are available), that you're not properly dressed for an interview. If the person feels comfortable with your casual attire—and is certain the interviewer won't hold it against you—don't let it shake your confidence. To be on the safe side, however, make a point to mention to the interviewer that you don't normally dress so informally for such important meetings.

We'd Like You to Meet the Company President

Somebody out there liked you because you've been asked back to meet an important muckity-muck. What to wear? Certainly something different from what you wore the first time, even if you just change your shirt and accessories. Ideally, you'll have another appropriate suit or can afford to spring for one (once you're at a certain job level, this is a must). Your goal: basically, just an encore performance (hey, it worked once!). Though making some minor adjustments (a less stuffy tie or a tad shorter skirt) to make you fit in better with the corporate culture is acceptable. Just rein in any urges to wear something trendy or flashy—even if it's in keeping with the company culture. Remember, you're still an outsider, not part of the team.

You're Hired!

You shined at the interviews and got the job. So now what? Do you: (a) pack away the smart-looking suits that so impressed those higher up the chain of command, or (b) wear them—or other outfits that reflect the same level of professionalism—again and again?

Of course, you picked *b,* which is clearly the winning strategy. Unfortunately, many people don't follow their own best instincts. Consider this real-life experience.

A friend once hired a young woman for an entry-level position. She didn't have much in the way of experience, but boy, did she ever look the part during the interview—a crucial factor, since she would frequently be in the public eye. Well, imagine my friend's dismay when her new assistant began showing up to work wearing clingy, low-cut tops and other garb better suited to a nightclub. Though it was fashionable, it was too provocative for a work environment—and a far cry from the sophisticated suit she had worn to the interview. "I felt like she had put one over on me, and frankly, it made me distrustful of her throughout the rest our working relationship."

If this story rings any bells, you need to be aware that securing employment isn't an end unto itself. Once in a position, you need to live up to the way you dressed at the interview. While that doesn't necessarily mean always being in a suit and tie, it certainly means not doing a complete turnabout and dressing completely out of character for the environment. Especially after presenting yourself well enough to get the job,

159

allowing your appearance to slide is a sure sign that something is amiss—either you don't take the position seriously, or you misrepresented yourself to get it. Either way, you'll certainly sabotage any chance of advancement.

The Least You Need to Know

➤ An interviewer's impression of you is formed within the first few seconds of your meeting. From then on, practically everything you do will be interpreted in such a way as to strengthen that initial impression.

➤ To convey respect for the importance of the interview, dress in a professional and respectful manner. Depending on your industry, this translates into wearing a suit or smart separates.

➤ When in doubt about what's appropriate to wear for an interview, always err on the conservative side. Sometimes that will require some compromise of your personal style and expression.

➤ Dressing appropriately for an interview requires thought and preparation. Never try to wing it the morning of the interview.

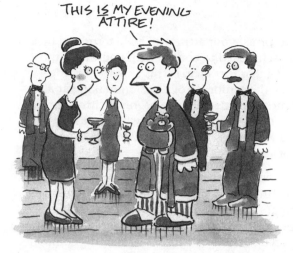

THIS IS MY EVENING ATTIRE!

Chapter 13

Out of the Office, but Still on the Job

In This Chapter

➤ Looking sharp at business meetings

➤ Meeting and eating

➤ Get a good reception

➤ Conventional wisdom

➤ Picnic apparel

➤ Party time

No matter how you normally dress for work, some situations—picnics, parties, receptions, meetings with business associates—will require a shift from the security of your everyday dress code into uncharted territory. Fear not, though! All will go smoothly once you realize that though these occasions may be fun, festive and held in far-flung places, they're still work-related affairs—and, as outlined in this chapter, require suitable professional attire.

Meeting Material

Meetings have a rap as being great time wasters ("they're indispensable when you don't want to do anything," wrote economist John Kenneth Galbraith), but it's hard to escape them. Easier is learning how to dress appropriately for one, to maximize both your confidence and the impression you make in these often high-pressure settings.

Meet the Requirements

Just as meetings can take many shapes and forms, your attire will be determined by a myriad of factors—including whom you're scheduled to confab with and the purpose of the meeting. For instance, is this a mettle-testing moment with the senior VP of decision making at a company whose business you've been soliciting for months, or a brainstorming session with your firm's public relations manager to strategize on building awareness of a new product?

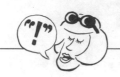

Quote . . . Unquote

You do so many things by phone and fax that you may only meet with a client three times a year. But when you do, you'd better be dressed appropriately. ...advertising agency president

According to one seasoned executive, dressing appropriately for meetings requires that you "take a pulse on the level of formality. If you have an in-house meeting, it's usually expected that the dress can be more relaxed than when you have outside visitors or are meeting someone on their own turf."

Even at Nike, a company that many consider to be the epitome of casual, it's not all sneakers and sweat suits. "It depends on the magnitude of the visitor, but generally our formality will be equal to his," says one employee, noting that, for example, a visit by the chairman of Nike Japan would certainly warrant a suit.

Still, no matter who you're meeting with, you want to be dressed in a fashion that boosts your confidence and ensures that you're taken seriously. "Because the senior sales manager is a very intimidating woman, I take extra care to be dressed like I know what I'm talking about during our weekly meeting. The confidence that gives me definitely has an effect on how poised I am during my presentation," says one account manager. Likewise, an executive in the pharmaceutical industry notes that when she attends a meeting in which she'll be the only woman, "I pick something that commands respect and keeps me on a level playing field with the men."

Stay a Step Above

No matter if they're on your turf or you're on theirs, when you have more riding on the outcome of the meeting, the practice of meeting or exceeding the expectations of the presentee should be standard operating procedure. "If you're trying to make a sale or to work in a more collaborative way, I expect you to dress as I am dressed, if not more formally—*you* are presenting to *me*," says one executive, who finds from her own experience that even if you develop different perceptions of people as you spend more time with them, that first impression is often how they'll be pegged.

The idea is to have your attire send the message that you've made an extra effort because this meeting holds special importance for you—that it's not something that happens every day. Such was the goal for the staff of a satellite office of a large corporation. "When we met with the officers of the company, a very wealthy contingent, we were expected to dress as if we just walked off a New York runway. I was always hyper about dressing well when they were in town because they were paying my salary."

Don't Be a Showoff

What requires some finesse is patterning your dress so that those with whom you're meeting don't look underdressed—or worse, feel that you're trying to show them up. "If you're calling on a client or potential client where the norm is to wear uniforms, goggles, and steel-reinforced shoes, you'd not only look out of place in a traditional business suit, you'd risk appearing condescending," notes a corporate vice president.

Fashion Footnote

According to estimates, the average executive spends over three hours a week in formal meetings and another eight in the more informal variety.

While it's sometimes difficult to exactly hit the mark (and nerve-wracking to try and psyche out the situation), the effort can pay dividends. As one sales rep, who had to determine a suitable outfit when calling on retailers in a rural community, states, "To them, it was a sign of respect, that, boy, you must think we're important!" For an attorney from a metropolitan area who's trying a case in an agricultural area, how he's dressed can even have an impact on the outcome of the trial. "Looking like the big-city hired gun can really backfire on you."

A logical tact is to look as people expect you to, but try and blend in a bit—whether that means trading in your suit for a smart sport jacket and slacks, or even wearing a pair of cowboy boots with your Brooks Brother's suit. "Making small accommodations can make you feel more comfortable in a new environment, and help others to feel more comfortable working with you," explains a fundraiser.

The Fashion Police

A smart strategy: "If I've met with someone once before, I note what they're wearing and then dress accordingly the next time," reports one executive. "If they're a bad dresser, I tend to dress down so there's not a huge contrast between the two of us."

Dressing for Dining

Business is often conducted over a meal. "You don't have to be in the office to do business. I've made so much money between courses," notes one businessman. To make it go off without a hitch, heed a few warnings. For instance, men, if you're unfamiliar with the restaurant where you'll be dining, call ahead to determine if it has a dress code. Some restaurants require men to wear a jacket, others a jacket and tie; unless you want to wear something of the management's choosing, check it out ahead of time.

You'll also want to think carefully about what to order. Some foods can be tricky to eat without draping yourself in a napkin, or leaving your hands—and potentially your whole outfit—a greasy mess, and as such, should be avoided in a business setting. (Soup, hard-to-handle pasta, crab legs, and triple-decker sandwiches fall into this category.) While it is considered correct for men to slip their ties into their shirts while eating, tucking a napkin into the neck of your shirt never is. On a similar note, dangling beads and long scarves, which can easily land on a woman's plate, aren't the best accessories at mealtime.

Finally, if you're wearing a heavy coat (or are carrying a number of packages), deposit the load with the coat-check attendant before greeting your dining partner. The tight quarters around restaurant tables don't usually permit much more than a purse or briefcase. Plus, it makes a better impression to walk in ready to shake hands with your dining companion.

Working the Room

As one of the single best opportunities for meeting new people and reconnecting with those you haven't seen in a while, a reception is a gathering with great potential for career advancement. "Employers are always on the lookout for talented new blood and this type of social situation allows them to scope things out in a friendly and relaxed manner," notes one CEO. On the flip side, a reception is the ideal occasion for you to win an introduction to a retailer to whom you are anxious to show your product—or at the very least, to meet someone who knows someone who knows the guy.

Considering the possibilities to see and be seen, you'll want to give some careful thought to the image you want to project to a roomful of people—many of whom you may not know. Of course, you'll want to wear something that makes you look and feel like a winner, so that you're teeming with self-confidence. Beyond that, you need to decide if you want to come across as serious and solid, original and creative, or something in between.

Your decision will depend on your profession and the goal you hope to accomplish—be it making a new contact or cultivating an existing relationship. For instance, is the event being held by a hip ad agency to introduce its new creative director—to whom you'd like to show your portfolio? Then by all means wear something stylish that marks you as a creative thinker. But if you're off to the annual meeting of the local bar association, stick with something more sartorially sedate—especially if you'll likely run into the managing partner of a firm that's considering you for an associate position.

Whatever you're wearing, a reception is an occasion at which you'll want to have business cards at the ready, either in your pocket or in a card case that's easily accessible—you don't want to be fumbling through your wallet or purse at every turn. One editor makes sure she wears a jacket with two pockets to receptions, one to hold her business cards, the other to stash any new cards she receives. "The last thing I want to do is mix the two together and run the risk of giving someone I've just met my last encounter's card!"

While we're on the subject of business cards, make sure that yours aren't half-torn, coffee-stained or out-of-date—with the wrong phone number or address on them. Now that you can get business cards printed overnight for a nominal amount of money, there's no excuse for presenting a card that's in anything other than mint condition.

Fashion Footnote

Think about how long you'll be standing at a reception and choose your shoes accordingly. You don't want to be chatting with a potential client when all you can think about is how pinched your toes are.

Trade Shows, Conventions, Sales Meetings, and Conferences

At some point in the course of your career, you'll likely be asked to pack a bag and head off to an industry gathering (for instance, a trade show or convention) or a company-sponsored event (like a sales meeting). If you're lucky, it will be held some-place warm and sunny and, more importantly, a dress code will have been announced in advance (oftentimes smaller conventions are declared business casual). If not, how you should dress will depend on a number of factors. Here are a few to consider:

➤ **The location**—Your attire will hinge somewhat on where you're going to be—whether it's a dude ranch in Wyoming, a lodge in Aspen, or a convention center in San Antonio. While you can use the destination to derive some cues as to the level of formality required of your dress, keep in mind that wardrobe protocol must be observed in even the most casual settings. So, in other words, leave the faded jeans and T-shirts at home.

➤ **Your role**—If you're going to be manning your company's booth at an annual trade show, it's not uncommon for a directive to be issued as to how employees should be dressed. More and more frequently, they're required to wear a "uniform." For instance, this year the convention crew at a computer company will be outfitted in navy blue sweaters, khaki pants, light colored shirts, and loafers. A similar outfit is worn by the sales staff of a flooring company. If, on the other hand, you're a buyer attending the show, dressing in close approximation to your normal business attire will help you establish your authority and communicate to vendors that you should be taken seriously. If casual is your company's dress code, now is the time to dust off your blazer and see to it that your shoes are shined—these types of meetings are ideal occasions to make a good impression on industry colleagues.

➤ **The itinerary**—Sometimes conferences span a number of days, and are planned so that there are business seminars or meetings during the day and dressier events at night. It can be tricky to plan for these meetings, since you'll be seeing the same people every day and will need clothes for a variety of situations. So that you'll have exactly what you'll need, but won't need five suitcases to fit it all, check out Chapter 15, "On the Road," for tips on planning a travel wardrobe.

The Company Picnic

You'd think that dressing for a picnic would be a snap, but when your boss—and his or her boss— will be in attendance, it's not always so simple. Sure, you know not to wear that barely decent pair of cutoffs or, since you will be seeing most of the people in attendance come Monday morning, anything else this side of scandalous. Along the same lines, you wouldn't be caught dead in something that could suggest that you don't know how to relax and have a little fun—like, say, a tie or pumps. But beyond that, you're just not sure how dressy to dress.

The first thing to know is where this shindig is being held: at a public park or the boss's country club? What activities are planned—softball? volleyball? tennis? golf? swimming? (This last nut has its own section.) What's on the menu? Is there a barbecuing committee, or is it being catered? All of these answers provide clues to the dress code.

The bottom line, however, is that even at their most formal, company outings should always be considered informal—and clothing along the lines of khakis and a sports shirt is about as dressy as it gets. If a fancier dinner is planned in the evening, be sure to bring a change of clothes—still on the sporty side, but a step up from the shorts you were wearing when you slid into third base.

Getting in the Swim of Things

It's the bane of most men's and women's company-picnic experience: having to wear a swimsuit. The $64,000 question is, Do I have to go swimming? In a word, no. "As self-conscious as I might be not swimming, I'd be that much more if all my lumps and bumps were on display for all my co-workers to see," declares one woman. If that's how your feel, no problem. Just sit on the sidelines sipping lemonade, outfitted in a tank suit with a pretty sarong or trunks and a T-shirt, if it makes you feel more a part of the aqueous action.

Should you choose to take the plunge, know that now is not the time to wear that thong bikini or your teeny Speedo. Even if you're in tremendous physical shape, anything too revealing may make an impression that you might later regret. Along the same lines, consider donning a cover-up of some kind in between dips; a tunic or even a big shirt will help you maintain modesty.

After Hours

Business often becomes social, and even if it happens only once a year—that is, the company Christmas party—it's important to know how to pull it off with panache.

9 to After 5

Whether you're going straight from work to the company bash or an industry cocktail party, you're after an evening look that's slightly festive, but not flashy.

Men can accomplish this simply: Wear a black or dark suit to work, and carry and change into a crisp white shirt with French cuffs and cuff links and a tie with a bit more sparkle—for instance, one with a slight sheen or iridescence. A pocket square and newly shined shoes complete the picture.

For women, a silky tank or lace camisole under the jacket beautifully alters the mood of a suit, as does a challis shawl over a coatdress. You can add some p.m. polish by substituting a velvet or satin top for your suit jacket and shirt. Accessories that work day and night: shiny croco-print or patent pumps and handheld purses, sheer or nude hose. A bulky shoulder bag—or worse, a briefcase!—and opaque hosiery are dead giveaways that you've come straight from the office. Illuminate your face with earrings and a necklace that catches the light.

After-hours makeup requires just five simple steps—not a complete overhaul:

1. To refresh foundation and give skin a dewy finish, lightly mist face with water. (The alternative, putting on powder, can leave skin looking cakey.)

2. Line upper eyelids with a smoky shade of eye shadow, pencil, or liner; turn up the line slightly at corners to lift eyes.

3. Brush a bit more blush on the apples of the cheek.

4. Apply a brighter or deeper shade of lipstick and top with gloss for added shine.

5. If you have another minute, curl eyelashes and/or add a second coat of mascara to open up eyes even more.

The Fashion Police

It's good policy to brush your teeth and freshen your breath before appearing in public. You don't want your otherwise impeccable appearance to be eclipsed by dragon breath or a leftover morsel of the muffin that you had for breakfast, do you?

To dress up hair, arrange longer locks in a French twist or neat bun, or add a pretty hairpin. Shorter hair can also look special: Add some gel to damp hair and sweep it back with a wide toothed comb for a textured, yet tailored look.

A Formal Affair

For most of us, it doesn't get any more formal than black-tie events, where tuxedos and longish dresses are de rigueur. (In actuality, however, white-tie is the ultimate in formality.) Hence formal affairs have the ability to scare even the best-dressed professional. The following guidelines will fill you with confidence.

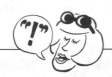

Quote . . . Unquote

My basic rules are to have shirt cuffs extend $1/2$ inch from the jacket sleeve. Trousers should break just above the shoe. Pocket handkerchiefs are optional, but I always wear one, usually orange, since orange is my favorite color. Shine your Mary Janes on the underside of a couch cushion. ...Frank Sinatra, on wearing a tux

Unlike women, who fret endlessly over their frocks, men have no choice as to their outfits for a black-tie soiree. A standard now for nearly a century, the tuxedo—which is named after Tuxedo Park, the city in New York where the first tuxedo-like jacket was worn to a formal ball—is both an ensemble of traditional uniformity and a suit capable of many looks. Here's how to pull off the polished look you desire.

Tux Tips:

➤ If renting a tuxedo, go to a shop that offers the greatest selection of designer suits and then pay whatever it takes to have the tux altered to fit you to a T. You want it to look as though you own it, not like it's a rental. This may take some legwork, but it can and should be done. Look through bridal magazines, which run scads of ads of tuxedos—including slightly more expensive brands that, when properly fitted, make you look anything but like a guy going to the prom.

➤ Tuxedo trousers shouldn't have cuffs, but should always have a stripe that matches the fabric of the jacket lapels running the entire length of the outside of the leg.

➤ Cummerbunds should be worn with single-breasted jackets, with the pleats facing upward. (In case you were wondering, their original purpose was to stash theater tickets.) Because double-breasted jackets stay buttoned, they don't require a cummerbund. A newer alternative to the cummerbund is a vest, which allows you remove your jacket and not look like a guy wearing a tux who took off his coat.

➤ Instead of black (which reportedly can take on a green tinge in certain lighting), consider opting for a midnight blue tuxedo, which is said to look blacker than black at night.

➤ The bow tie should match or go well with the fabric of your jacket lapels. It doesn't have to be solid black, however; gold, silver, or a tasteful pattern in rich colors and fabrics can set a man apart from the penguin pack.

➤ Don't try to distinguish yourself via your shirt, at least if you're thinking ruffles or turquoise trim. Stick with a classic white shirt with a straight or wing-tip collar and, of course, French cuffs.

➤ Always hand tie your bow tie. A clip-on is déclassé. (See Chapter 9, "Accessories: Special Effects," for how-tos.)

➤ Do not buy or rent the shoes with bows. Go with a simple cap-toe dress shoe. Nonviable options are your everyday wing-tips or any casual shoe that will spoil the dressy effect.

Fashion Footnote

Why rent when you can own? If you go to two formal functions a year, it pays to buy a tuxedo. When and if you do, choose the most enduring style—that is, single-breasted with a notched or shawl collar.

For women, black-tie doesn't necessarily translate into a black dress—or even a dress for that matter. An evening jacket or elegant blouse paired with a long, black velvet or satin skirt or trousers can look just as luxurious. Compared to an unforgettable dress, which—if you usually travel in the same circles—may only get one go-round, separates offer glamour and versatility. Bright colors and bold patterns are equally appropriate (and even more dramatic), but necessitate quieter accessories than, say, a simple black sheath, which can withstand more adornment.

When choosing your attire, aim to look sophisticated rather than sexy; clothing that's flimsy or resembles lingerie is best saved for purely social events. What about going sleeveless or choosing an outfit with some "northern exposure?" If you've got great arms, a sleeveless dress or blouse isn't too risqué, provided that the rest of the garment is conservatively styled; if it's also backless or designed with a thigh-high slit, you'd do best to choose something less racy. Anything more revealing, like, say, a strapless dress, could also be trouble, especially if the fit isn't perfect. "There tends to be lots of hugging and dancing at these events," notes an executive who frequently attends such doings. "You don't want to risk anything falling out."

"If you're the host or a participant in the evening's festivities, choosing appropriate attire requires that much more consideration," notes a woman who emcees her organization's black-tie fundraiser every year. "This event is a huge thing for us, and I need to feel very confident in my appearance. Since I'll be running around all night, I look for something I can move in comfortably. I can't be worried about tripping on my dress." In her experience an ankle-length garment is easiest to get around in.

169

When dressed to the nines, do not neglect what you're wearing over your dress or tux. For a woman, a regular wool coat will ruin the effect; instead, wrap yourself up in a silky shawl—or one that looks like cashmere. For men, a dark, classically styled coat is the perfect topper.

The Fashion Police

Women, for a formal or semiformal affair, you may want to rethink wearing a slip dress; oftentimes flimsy and similar to lingerie, slip dresses may be too sexy for work affairs. Save them for special occasions when you're on your own time.

"Creative" Black Tie

Don't be surprised when an invitation arrives that specifies dress as creative black tie. The latest craze in formal attire, creative black tie is simply a way of indicating that while the affair will be a dressy one, guests can feel free to be a bit more expressive with their attire—something that has more meaning for men than women, who already have a lot of latitude with evening dress. Just don't take the directive too far: Think more along the lines of substituting a tartan cummerbund for a black one, less about pairing your hightops and your tux.

The Fashion Police

What's appropriate for a semiformal event? Semiformal functions usually require a fairly dressy suit, dress, or pants outfit—in any length or color. Men can get by with a dark suit and dressier accessories. When in doubt, ask for details when you RSVP.

The Least You Need to Know

➤ Not all work is conducted in your office, your building, or between the hours of nine and five. Even if the occasion seems social, it's important to maintain a professional appearance.

➤ How to dress for a meeting is determined by whom the meeting is with and by where and why it's being held. Whatever your personal mode of dress, it's best to alter it so that you meet expectations of the other party.

➤ When meeting a business associate for a meal, inquire ahead of time as to the restaurant's dress code.

➤ The appropriate dress for a reception depends on the impression you wish to make on the other people in attendance. Whatever your attire, be sure to have on hand enough business cards so that you can offer one as needed.

➤ How you should dress for out-of-town meetings will depend on where they're being held, your assigned role, and the scheduled itinerary.

➤ Although a company picnic is a time to relax and enjoy the company of your co-workers, it's inappropriate to wear your shortest shorts, muscle-man T-shirt, or teeny, weeny bikini.

➤ Industry functions afford you the opportunity to demonstrate your social skills, as well as your fashion refinement.

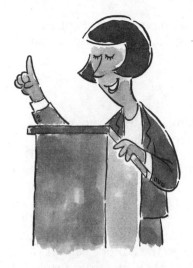

When All Eyes Are on You

If you've never appeared on television, spoken before a large crowd, or had your picture professionally taken, take my word for it, the experience can run the emotional gamut from nerve-wracking to downright terrifying.

My first TV experience was a national news program that was taped live, meaning there was no chance for a second "take" if I flubbed an answer. Even though the general reaction to my performance was quite positive, those five minutes of fame were enough for a lifetime, and I swore I'd never do TV again. But, for one reason or another, I got roped into doing publicity more times than I cared to oblige—and each time I picked up additional tidbits of information on dressing and grooming that helped me appear more telegenic on each subsequent appearance.

Since, like me, you probably don't earn your living by being photographed, or appearing on TV or in front of podiums, you may never have pondered your public image. But when the opportunity arises for your 15 minutes of fame—be it via an invitation to speak in front of 100 colleagues, an appearance on a local television show, or a photo in the community newspaper—you want to be able to accept the offer knowing that your efforts to get some good publicity won't be canceled out by a bad appearance. It's when you need to present a flattering and professional public persona that the information in this chapter will come in handy.

Picture Perfect

A picture can be worth *more* than a thousand words (and none of them very good) if it's on display and your outfit begs for unflattering commentary. But with these pointers, looking good will be a snap—even if the photo is just for your company I.D. card.

Dressing for Your Close-Up

When you're going to be photographed, dress in comfortable clothing that reflects the image you're trying to project. For instance, in her picture on the Editor's Page of *Redbook,* then-editor-in-chief Kate White wore a stylishly serious, butter-colored suit, an outfit that, while befitting her position as the top editor of a national magazine, also made her look approachable and friendly—an understandable goal when you're trying to reach out and touch your readers.

For similar reasons, Dan Rather—who was viewed as being too stiff after taking over for Walter Cronkite—often softens his image by wearing a sweater under his suit, or losing the jacket altogether, when going before a camera.

On the other hand, when you see official pictures of most captains of industry, they're usually dressed conservatively, in dark suits and light-colored shirts that create an aura of authority. That there's little doubt they're in charge of something is precisely the look they're going for!

Whatever message you're trying to send, wear an outfit in a simple, timeless style—anything fussy or busy including patterns, will divert attention from your image. Do, however, consider wearing something with a nubby texture, rather than say a flat wool or silk jacket—to provide some visual interest. (Don't confuse a pebbly surface with an overpowering pattern, like houndstooth check or windowpane plaid.) For a professional portrait, you want to be wearing a jacket—or a suit if the photo will show you full figure. It will provide the most streamline look. Some other tips:

Fashion Footnote

Try to schedule your photo session at least a week after getting a haircut, so that you don't have that new-haircut look.

Fashion Footnote

Keep in mind that you may need to use the same photo 5 years, even 10 years, from when it's taken. If you're dressed in a trendy outfit or color, the photo will instantly be dated (even if you're not!).

➤ Tuck shirts into hose or underwear to prevent bunching.

➤ Sit on coattails to keep your jacket from riding up in back.

➤ Check your posture. People often slouch when being photographed, either because that's their natural stance or because they'd rather be anywhere other than in front of a camera getting their picture taken.

➤ Think about your feet. If they're going to be in the photo, your socks should match your pants or shoes, and your shoes must be clean and presentable.

Color Me Photogenic

Unless you're being photographed by Richard Avedon or Francesco Scavullo for *Vanity Fair*, don't wear all black or all white—neither of which photographs well. Black absorbs color and obliterates any detail. It will likely make you look as though your head isn't anchored to your body. White reflects light and "blows out," causing the same problem. Your head will look as if it's mounted on a light bulb, and your complexion will be completely pale to boot.

Now that you know the don'ts, here are the do's to looking professional in a picture.

➤ Consider carefully what message you want your clothing to convey. Bright colors will make you appear energetic; dark colors, more authoritative. Discuss your options with the photographer, who can help guide you. Always safe is a medium- or dark-colored jacket, paired with a light-colored shirt. (It's for this reason that a dark jacket and light blue shirt combination is so popular for pictures). Light-colored jackets are generally not good choices, as they don't frame your face and can wash you out. Use a tie or scarf to add a splash of color.

➤ Wear a color that you feel good in and that flatters your complexion and hair color. (Refer to Chapter 10, "So Many Options!" for further information.) Especially if you're tired or feeling under the weather, wear something bright near your face to give it some color.

➤ Avoid too much white near your face, unless it's offset with a scarf, necklace, or necktie.

➤ Dress monochromatically, if your entire body will show. A light top and dark bottom will cut you in half and make you appear shorter and fatter, while the reverse will make you look like a pear! Shoulder-to-ankle in the same shade makes for the cleanest, longest line. If you're wearing a skirt, however, don't try to match your hose; nude-colored hosiery looks best in a photo.

Keep It Simple

Wear few, if any, accessories. Belts, scarves, earrings, necklaces, bracelets, rings, and watches are fine, but don't wear them altogether. A good rule is to pick three that make sense (a belt, earrings, and watch, or scarf, earrings, and bracelet, for example). If you have a tendency to overdo it, follow Mary Lou Henner's lead in the film *L.A. Story*: Stand in front of a mirror, quickly look away, and look back. Take off the first thing you see. It's usually an accessory screaming out.

The Fashion Police

Should you have your photo re-touched? Absolutely. While you don't want to airbrush yourself to death, the softening of some lines and the lightening of dark areas can help you project a more pleasing image.

Putting Your Best Face Forward

If you've ever seen celebrities pose for candid shots, you know that they're very good at instantly positioning themselves for the most flattering photo. (Watching a renown physician remove her glasses, cock her head to the left, and smile demurely in one motion when a camera came into view once left me totally mesmerized!) So that you can feel more at ease and look your best in photos, spend some time in front of the mirror getting comfortable with your image and then have a friend snap a few photos of you sometime so you can experiment with different angles. While you're practicing, try incorporating these tricks of the trade:

➤ **Weak chin?** Tilt your head and lower your chin. Self-conscious about a double chin? De-emphasize it by raising your chin, and turning your face slightly to the right or left (depending on which profile you prefer) while still looking into the camera.

➤ **Too many facial lines?** Ask the photographer to surround you with bright light—a trick employed by age-conscious actors and actresses.

➤ **Don't like your smile?** Think happy thoughts or about someone you love. Even though your mouth isn't smiling, your eyes will be. The twinkle in them and the generally happy look on your face will make you look pleasant.

➤ **Bothered by under-eye circles?** Conceal darkness, which can be exaggerated with harsh lighting, with a cover-up cream that matches your foundation. Apply eye shadow and mascara only to upper lids and lashes to avoid adding more darkness to the area below. Lifting your chin will also make dark circles look less so.

➤ **Nose too prominent?** If your nose looks big to you in pictures, it may be because you're dropping your chin. Try lifting it up instead.

➤ **Want to accentuate your eyes?** Drop your chin and look directly into the camera.

➤ **Worried about helmet hair?** Hair should be styled as you wear it naturally, with just a bit more oomph or polish. Too much gel or spray in your hair can zap its natural body and shine. Very thick hair can benefit from strategically placed hair color highlights, which add definition. Placing the lightest shades in the front will frame your face with lightness. Don't forget to have your roots touched up; they will photograph darker than they really are.

➤ **Nervous?** The camera will pick up your mood, so don't start until you feel completely comfortable. Taking deep breaths can relieve tension in you face and body. Talking to the photographer also often helps make you feel more at ease.

When it comes to makeup, it's well worth the investment to hire a professional makeup artist. If you can't afford one, heed this important advice.

➤ Don't pile on the paint. Too much makeup is the most common mistake. Makeup should be used sparingly and with care, so it makes you look like the best possible version of yourself. Generally, it's best to go with a slightly enhanced version of your natural makeup.

➤ Apply makeup in natural light. Makeup artists work with the photographer so they know what the light is going to look like. Since you won't, it's safest to work near a window.

Fashion Footnote

When being photographed, position yourself at a three-quarter angle, which is the most flattering view. No one looks good photographed from below.

➤ Make sure your foundation is a good match for your complexion. One that's too light looks especially "pasty" in a photograph.

➤ To control shine, dust on power that exactly matches your skin tone with a puff.

➤ Don't use bronzing powder, since any orangey undertones will be exaggerated on film. If you think you look too pale, use powder a touch darker than your normal foundation.

Black, White, and Professional All Over

Black-and-white photographs pose some special problems. Though the format has perhaps the greatest potential for drama, generally speaking, a person who needs a

Fashion Footnote

To reacquaint yourself with how colors look in black and white, turn down the color on your TV while watching your favorite show.

photo to send with a bio or to include on a business card wants to look credible, confident, and sincere—not overly dramatic.

Toward this end, you'll definitely want to stay away from all black or all white outfits; middle tones together with lighter and darker accents can provide contrast and interest without dramatic overkill. Remember that every color translates to a shade of gray in black-and-white photos, meaning you'll want to go for tonal contrast, not color contrast. For instance, a red and a blue that contrast sharply when photographed in color may translate as two similar values of gray in black and white. Again, consult the photographer for professional advice.

Makeup-wise, use a light hand and neutral colors; dark lipstick, for instance, photographs as black.

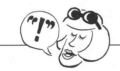

Quote . . . Unquote

If you look like your passport photo, you're too ill to travel. ...Will Kommen

Lights, Camera, Action!

In this day of network and cable talk shows, news magazines, business programs, panel discussions, and national and local news, the chance that you might someday be asked to make an appearance on the small screen is growing. (The trend toward videoconferencing will further increase this possibility.) Considering the high stakes, and the fact that everything is magnified on the screen, some preparation for the camera is crucial. Here are some good starting points:

➤ Preview the program on which you'll be appearing, so that you dress appropriately. For instance, if you'll be discussing emerging markets on the *Bloomberg Business Report*, you'll want to look like the businessmen and businesswomen who are probably tuning in. Conversely, if you're going to be featured in a segment on a lifestyle program showing the best Christmas presents for under $50 (a gig I once had), it's not necessary to look all buttoned up.

➤ Find out in advance if you'll be sitting or standing, the latter position poses less potential problems. If you're going to be seated, be extremely conscious of your posture, since even a little slump can create shadows in the creases of your shirt or jacket. Sit straight, but not in such an exaggerated manner that you look stiff. Many experts advise that women wear pants. "When you wear a skirt, you're busy wondering if it's all the way up your leg. Pants give you one less thing to worry about," notes a media trainer. If you're planning on wearing a skirt, check

ahead of time in a mirror that it's long
enough to cover your thighs when you're
seated. While you're at it, see how you look
with your legs crossed; frankly, many
women don't have the legs to pull it off and
would be wiser to keep them together,
crossed at the ankles.

➤ Consider whether your hands will be on
display. Before filming the Christmas gift
spot, in which my hands were on view at
least half the time, I scheduled a manicure.
You may want to consider doing the same,
especially if you naturally gesture a lot—
which can draw attention to your hands.

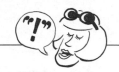

Quote . . . Unquote

I have great legs, so I'm always
looking to show them off. But I
don't wear short skirts on our TV
show "The View" because there's a
time and place for everything. The
last thing I want is my skirt hiking
up, making me look awkward and
flustered. ...Star Jones, in her book,
*You Have to Stand for Something,
or You'll Fall for Anything*

The Fashion Police

Even if a particular garment is otherwise ideal for on-air wear, avoid wearing it if it's too
tight. Anything snug can inhibit your breathing, and shallow breathing can make you feel
stressed.

Tips for Looking Telegenic

The same rules of color, silhouette, and accessories apply. Whether you're being
broadcast to millions or having your meeting videotaped. With these cameras, however, lights are much brighter, and movement and sound are also factors.

Wear Solids

Stripes, unless bold or finer and spaced far apart, are absolutely taboo, since they
appear to move and smear on film. Large or busy patterns scream for attention, and
small prints may morph into a distracting blur. Check ahead with the production crew
for suggestions on color; their advice will take into consideration the background of
the set, into which you don't want to fade. Some colors that generally don't work on
TV: red, which has the tendency to create a halo effect, and any hue so bright that it

might visually assault the viewer. And no matter how much you fear the 10 pounds that TV adds, don't dress in all black: it's absolutely deadening on camera.

Avoid Fussy or Oversized Accessories

Jewelry should be minimal. A superchunky necklace could look like a noose, as was the case one night when Barbara Walters wore a beautiful, but gigantic necklace on *20/20*. After the program, the 11 o'clock news announcers in Los Angeles commented relentlessly on its size. Also skip large, loose bracelets and dangling earrings; they tend to move and clank. As for glasses, many of the newer styles don't reflect light as much as the older types, but they still might present lighting difficulties because of the potential to cast shadows. In addition, they form a barrier between you and your audience. If possible, wear contacts, or if you can get by without the glasses (and you don't have a tendency to squint), consider taking them off for the cameras. Definite don'ts are half-glasses or those that are tinted or light sensitive.

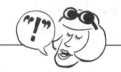

Quote . . . Unquote

There were complaining phone calls because you were sweating? No, nice ones, worried that I was having a heart attack. ...Holly Hunter's character to Albert Brooks' character in *Broadcast News*

Wear a Jacket

A jacket helps hide rolls and paunches offers a clean, powerful silhouette, and provides lapels for microphones and coverage for hidden wires. Oftentimes a microphone box will be clamped to your waistband in back, so be sure there's at least an inch of space to accommodate it.

Makeup Is a Must

Yes, even for men! Lights give off heat that cause the skin to perspire (a natural reaction that viewers may interpret negatively), so at the very least allow your face to be powdered.

For women, the ideal TV face should be a natural, everyday face, just more defined and vivid. Most TV programs will have a makeup artist on staff. If not, and you have to do it yourself, simply add a bit more blush to counteract the paling effect of bright lights (blend well to avoid the look of war markings), a fresh application of lipstick (stay with a matte finish, as going glossy can make you look like a starlet), and oil-absorbing powder to your regular makeup.

For those women who normally go without, here's the on-camera minimum:

➤ Foundation that matches and blends into your jaw line (at the very least, cover blemishes, any discolorations, and under-eye circles).

➤ Blush applied to the apples of your checks and out toward the hairline (without it your face may appear flat and one dimensional).

➤ A neutral rose, pink, or peach lipstick (avoid reds and bright pinks, which will jump out at the camera, and browns and purples, which may make your mouth look dull or ghoulish).

➤ Black mascara on top lashes only (bad lighting can cause tarantula-like shadows under the eyes).

➤ Plenty of oil-absorbing powder—whenever possible, use powder makeup, as creams can run under hot lights and collect in lines and creases.

This routine is much more modified—but no less essential—for men, who usually have blemishes covered, dark areas lightened, and shiny spots (including a thinning pate) powdered.

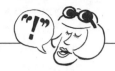

Quote . . . Unquote

Your personality should shine, not your face—or your lips or eyes, for that matter. The lights used when filming will reflect shine and make you look greasy. Wear plenty of face powder and avoid high-gloss lipsticks or sparkly, glimmery eyeshadow. ...New York City–based makeup artist Paula Dorf, who has worked with everyone from President Clinton to Cindy Crawford

Public Speaking: Shining in the Spotlight

If the mere thought of giving a speech makes you quiver, you're not alone. According to polls, Americans biggest fear is making a speech. Nothing surprising about that: Being in front of an audience has always been a double-edged sword. If all goes well, the exposure can be extremely valuable to your career and/or your cause. But with this increased ability to have others focus on you and your message, you're also inviting potential problems. The following guidelines will help ensure that you look as credible as you sound:

➤ **Wear clothing you feel comfortable in**—This is key to appearing at ease, since anything that binds, pinches, or is restrictive in any way will prevent you from moving freely and naturally. Body language is very important when you're speaking to a group; according to research, listeners base 55 percent of their reaction to a speaker on nonverbal factors, so you don't want to wear clothing that makes you feel self-conscious or look stiff or awkward. Again, if they'll be seated, women should consider wearing pants. "That way you're not worried as much about keeping your knees together," points out a women who frequently appears on panels.

➤ **Tailor your outfit to your audience and what they're likely to be wearing**—If you'll be lecturing to a group of doctors decked out in conservative business suits, sporting anything less formal will undermine your image. Even if you're a brilliant person with a riveting message, a strange or distracting appearance could convince your audience otherwise.

➤ **Choose confidence-boosting clothes**—A suit is always powerful, but any outfit that matches your audience and makes you feel in control is fine. Avoid scratchy wools or heavy fabrics such as cashmere or flannel. Since you may already be nervous, you don't want to increase your odds of dripping sweat. If you're worried about excessive perspiration, wear a lighter-colored suit, which may make it less noticeable.

➤ **If appropriate, wear color**—Bold colors will make you appear more dynamic, even if it's just a splash of red in a tie or a deep-blue shirt. They can also get you noticed. "I always wear red when I'm on a panel. You can't miss me, and then afterward if someone wants to meet me, I'm easy to spot in a sea of blue suits," says the president of a public relations firm. Plus, because you often stand in front of a dark background when speaking (frequently without a spotlight to illuminate you), you'll blend into the background otherwise. Skip obnoxious, loud shades (neons, fuchsia, and chartreuse, for example) or ostentatious patterns, which are distracting. "The goal is to have people notice that you look nice, not the fact that your suit is fuchsia," says a former lobbyist.

➤ **Be wary of pattern**—Many prints, plaids, and textures create optical illusions when viewed from afar. Stand as far away from a mirror as you can to determine what effect the audience will see.

➤ **Minimize accessories**—The elegant brooch styled like a lizard might look stunning up close, but confusing from 12 feet away. Don't keep your audience wondering what you're wearing throughout your presentation; the guessing game can be distracting, and, after all, you do want them to remember what you said, don't you? Also avoid clunky bracelets, flowing scarves, and shiny metals or stones that could catch the light. And instead of carrying your purse or briefcase to the stage, have someone you trust hold onto it.

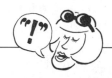

Quote . . . Unquote

The longest walk in the whole world is from the back of the conference room to the podium, so if women aren't confident in high heels, I advocate not wearing them. ...Joyce Newman, president of The Newman Group, a New York City–based firm specializing in media training

➤ **Empty your pockets**—Bulging pockets look odd and will distract the audience.

➤ **Don't forget your feet**—The audience will look up at them if you're on a stage, so make sure that your socks are high enough and that your shoes are clean and polished. Comfort is also key, especially if you'll be standing during your presentation. Most important, shoes should allow you to move quickly and confidently.

➤ **Check yourself out beforehand, top and bottom, front to back**—Even if you won't consciously turn your back to your audience, it may be in plain view as your approach and leave the podium. A full-length mirror works fine for this, but if you have access to video equipment, you may want to videotape a practice session during which you wear your planned outfit.

The Least You Need to Know

➤ Your public image can be a lasting one; dress in minimum-fuss clothes that fit well, make you feel confident, and keep the focus on your image or message.

➤ Always consider your audience and try to match its level of formality. When in doubt, suits are the safest, most powerful bet.

➤ Loud, big, bright, or sparkly accessories can cause technical havoc by creating glare or distracting sound when you're before a TV or video camera. Keep accessories to a minimum.

➤ Don't make any radical changes to your appearance just prior to being photographed or appearing publicly. If you're at all uncomfortable with the look, your discomfort will surely show.

➤ Real men wear makeup. Hot lights make you perspire, so—at the bare minimum—powder is a must.

➤ Before appearing in public, consider videotaping your presentation so you can assess you appearance from your audience's perspective. At the very least, have a dry-run the night before the big day, so you can preview your outfit and make any necessary adjustment.

Part 5
Special Conditions

At work, everything can change on a dime and undermine your steely dress-for-success resolve. Suddenly you're booked on the red-eye to the coast, with only two hours to pack and get to the airport. Or spring gives way to summer one June morning, leaving you to cope with 90-degree heat and humidity—plus the stress of the Jones deposition. Or the pregnancy that you're tickled pink (or blue) about but are trying to keep under wraps for another two weeks, is becoming more and more obvious every day.

It's for these career challenges, which can elevate your status or diminish it just as quickly, that this section was written. The information in Chapter 15, "On the Road," will help take the sartorial stress out of traveling, whether you're crossing the Atlantic on a week-long fact-finding mission or just crossing the state line to check out a snafu in a satellite office. To keep the weather from ruining your professional presentation, turn to Chapter 16, "The Weather Outside Is Frightful" and Chapter 17, "The Heat Is On." And to nip in the bud any doubt about your commitment to your career while pregnant, see Chapter 18, "From Here to Maternity."

In each of these chapters, you'll find sure-fire strategies for staying on the road to success, no matter how many speed bumps you encounter.

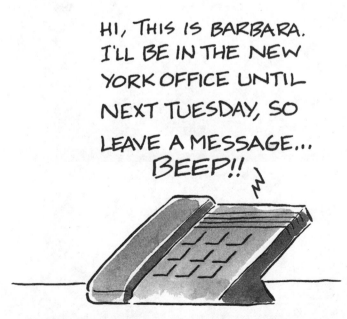

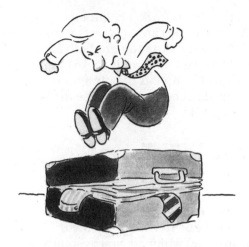

Chapter 15

On the Road

In This Chapter

➤ The lowdown on luggage

➤ Packing pointers

➤ Carry on?

➤ Dressing en route

➤ How do they dress there?

If you've traveled much for work, it probably won't surprise you to learn that the word travel is derived from the French term *travaillier*, which alternatively means to labor and torture. While those who don't go on the road much will probably never be convinced that traveling is anything but glamorous and exciting, the fact is that when you add tight scheduling, unfamiliar surroundings, and jet lag to the often uncomfortable means of getting where you're going, business travel is often more stressful than your regular work routine—even if you are in an exciting city or exotic country.

Still, because conferences, conventions, and presentations frequently mean travel, you'll be expected to look polished when conducting business in some faraway city and living out of a suitcase—a goal that's easily accomplished once you know some key things. For instance, just what passes as professional when you're in Russia, Rio, or whatever your final destination? How should you pack so that you're not so weighted down with suitcases that you look like a skycap—or so underpacked that you end up wearing the same suit for six days? What's appropriate attire while you're in transit?

Fashion Footnote

Generally, the upper limit for luggage to be stowed under the seat or overhead is 45 inches overall, when you add up the length, height, and depth of the bag. Be aware, however, that when flying on smaller aircraft, there's usually less space for carry-on bags.

Having logged a lot of miles for work, I count myself as something of an authority in this area. (In fact, at one point in my career, I traveled constantly, for both long and short stretches.) As a result, I not only racked up frequent-flyer points, I picked up lots of pointers on how to look your professional best while on the road—all of which are in this chapter.

Have Suitcase Will Travel

There's little doubt that your luggage is the linchpin in how professional you appear to be when traveling on business. No matter how sharply you're dressed, showing up at the airport laden down with unmatched, overstuffed, and/or ratty bags will mark you as someone who simply doesn't belong in business class (a distinction I don't necessarily mean literally). As airline attendants long ago figured out, the key to looking like a savvy traveler is to be in control of your luggage—rather than have it be in control of you.

Frankly, this is something I've had to learn the hard way, having struggled for years with no-frills bags that, though lightweight and durable, were still cumbersome to carry (absolute murder on the neck and shoulder!), and sadly lacking in any special features that would make packing less of a chore.

Fashion Footnote

If you're not in the market for new luggage but are tired of carrying your bag, spring for a luggage cart, a collapsible carrier that allows you to push or pull your luggage.

Today, there's little reason not to have luggage that both makes traveling easier and enhances your image. Precisely what type of luggage you'll want depends on several factors, including what you'll be packing. For example, duffle bags, which are often soft sided and frameless, are better suited to more casual clothing, while garment bags, which permit you to transport your garments on hangers, are ideal when carrying full-length clothes.

To determine what type of luggage will best serve your needs, scope out a luggage store—the options are mindboggling. Meanwhile, here's some background.

The Pullman

The rectangular case that has long been synonymous with the work suitcase, the pullman is the bag to have if you're only going to have one piece of luggage. Basically a box with a hinged lid, pullmans can accommodate everything a business traveler needs to have on hand—especially if you choose one with special compartments designed to hold your suits or dresses. (Such "suiters" are designed with padded bars or fabric straps that hold suits in place with limited folding, and subsequently, little creasing.)

A large percentage of pullmans now come equipped with wheels and "telescoping" handles, those that pull out and then disappear back into the suitcase and that let you steer with the touch of a finger. If you're a frequent flyer in the market for luggage, these two back-saving features are musts.

A Hard or Soft Shell

Pullmans come in two main constructions—hard and soft sided. Though the former (fashioned of hard plastic or metal) might have the edge in durability and resistance to crushing, the fact is that strong, yet lightweight materials (usually nylon or polyester), coupled with some partial frames or stiffeners to help them hold their shape, make soft-sided suitcases better at absorbing shocks when thrown around. They also make it easier to squeeze in one last thing when the bag is already overpacked!

Another significant consideration: The lightest soft-sided bag can weigh as little as one and a half pounds; a hard-sided suitcase can weigh 10 pounds empty.

Garment Bags

Available in a range of lengths (from 40 inches for suits to 60 inches for dresses and evening clothes), garment bags act as portable closets. There are two kinds: Garment covers, which are simple zippered sheaths, and more elaborate gusseted bags constructed of a soft material that's sometimes stretched on a frame. These have greater capacity (depending on the size, they're usually able to hold at least four garments) and, for easier carrying, can fold over. (If you choose a longer version, look for a bag that will fold into thirds, so as to fit under the seat or overhead). Like pullmans, some garment bags now also come on wheels and sport retractable handles.

Pack It In

Packing isn't just an art or a science, it's a bit of both. To do it successfully, you need to plan wisely (so you can keep suitcases to a minimum, yet have everything you need) and load up your luggage properly (to ensure that everything arrives safely and soundly with as few creases as possible).

Fashion Footnote

Denier is a numbering system in which low numbers represent fine yarn sizes and high numbers indicate coarser, heavier sizes—and consequently, stronger, more durable fabric. Ballistic nylon, which is over 1,000 denier, is so strong that perforations do not tear the fabric. The average business traveler, however, can usually survive quite nicely with luggage made of 420-denier nylon or 600-denier polyester.

The Fashion Police

Wildly colored and patterned luggage may be easy to spot on the baggage carousel, but carrying gear in neutral-colored and subtly patterned bags looks more professional. If you want to distinguish your bags, use colorful luggage tags.

Prepping Like the Pros

Before even thinking about packing, you must plan your wardrobe. To do this, you need to know your itinerary: where you'll be (Hawaii in July or Chicago in January?), how long you'll be there (just overnight or a full week?), and what you'll be doing (manning the company's booth at an international trade show or checking out construction on a new building designed by your firm?).

Once you know what's on the agenda, you can start planning your wardrobe. To limit how much you need to take, follow these guidelines:

➤ Pack around a color scheme that includes just two neutrals—for instance, beige and black or navy and gray. (If you've followed this advice in choosing your wardrobe, selecting your travel clothes should be easy.) This way, your shirts, sweaters, ties, and other accessories will all mix and match with your jackets and pants and/or skirts.

➤ If you must wear suits, determine how many times you'll see the same people and plan accordingly—bearing in mind that there's nothing wrong with wearing the same suit more than once (preferably with a day of rest in between wearings), provided you change the shirt and accessories.

➤ Choose clothes that can be worn in more than one way: The right jacket can accompany a coordinating skirt or pant during the day and dressier or more casual pieces in the evening.

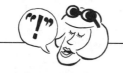

Quote . . . Unquote

A journey of 1,000 miles must begin with one step—packing. ...sixth century philosopher, Lao Tzu

Before packing everything into your suitcase, do what fashion editors do: Lay out all the pieces of each outfit on a flat surface (the bed is easier than the floor), grouped with the necessary accessories. This way, you can actually visualize each outfit and be sure you have all the pieces required to complete it.

190

The Fashion Police

If you pack 100 percent linen clothing for a business trip, you can be pretty certain, it will be a wrinkled mess by the time you arrive. Better options are knitted garments (cotton, wool, or synthetics) or those made of wool, silk, or synthetic fibers—which resist wrinkles and release them with relative ease. The most travel-friendly fabric? Wool and silk crepes, which are woven from naturally springy, high-twist yarns.

Packing 101

Careful packing can make the difference between clothes that look crumpled upon arrival and those that only need some touching up. A garment bag is a breeze to pack—just hang everything up, taking care to slip a plastic bag (like those you get from the dry cleaner) over the hanger, and then in between each layer of clothing. It's the pullman-style cases that require some counsel. Here are the ins and outs:

➤ Pack in layers. Everyone has their own system of packing, but if you don't have a "suiter" suitcase, I suggest a method of folding that ultimately creates an interwoven bundle of clothing, one that keeps garments from becoming crushed and wrinkled. Begin by placing on the bottom of the suitcase underwear, socks, and pajamas—anything that isn't affected by wrinkles. Pants go in next, draped so that the legs extend outside the bag (be sure pockets are empty, and that pants are zipped and folded along natural creases). Place sweaters, skirts, and dresses in next, arranging the waistbands or collars at the alternating edges of the suitcases, and allowing any surplus fabric to hang out on both sides. Once everything is in place, "interfold": alternating from side to side, fold the edges of one garment over the other—always taking care to smooth away wrinkles.

➤ Putting a piece of tissue or a plastic dry-cleaner wrapping between garments helps prevent creasing.

Fashion Footnote

To conserve space, wear, don't pack, the heavier clothes (and shoes) you're bringing while traveling. If you're traveling from a cold climate to a warm one, dress for arrival, not departure. You don't usually need an overcoat in Miami in January.

Fashion Footnote

Call ahead and ask what services the hotel offers. If speedy, reasonably priced, dry cleaning or laundry service is available, why pack more than two suits or three or four shirts? And if the hotel supplies hair dryers and irons (some store one of each in every room), why duplicate efforts? Ditto shampoo, conditioner, and soap—unless you have a real loyalty to your own brand.

➤ Before being packed, a jacket should be neatly folded. Flatten the sleeves lengthwise, and position diagonally toward the center of the jacket. Then fold the lower half of the jacket over the top, taking care to place another garment in between.

➤ Shirts that have been bagged and boxed at the laundry travel best. Otherwise, neatly fold sleeves, and position shirts so that they'll be folded below the waistline—where any creases will be out of site.

➤ Roll up ties to prevent wrinkling.

➤ If you don't use shoe trees, stuff socks into shoes— both to save space and protect the shoes. Pack shoes in plastic bags, old socks, or the felt pouches you can buy in stores, and place around the perimeter of your suitcase—heels facing outward.

➤ Carry toiletries in plastic bags, to prevent damage in the event of leakage. Sample sizes are real space savers. To prevent toiletries from bursting in flight, fill bottles partway, then squeeze out excess air, and seal to form a vacuum.

➤ If you're going some place where ironing won't be possible, know that it's hard to tell if a checked shirt is wrinkled.

➤ Above all else, pullmans should be packed snugly, so contents have less chance of shifting—and possibly wrinkling. (If you run out of room while packing, close the bag and drop it on the floor. Thing inside should settle, creating room for more.) Conversely, garment bags shouldn't be overstuffed, for the same reason.

To Check or Not To Check

Checking your luggage can certainly make your trip more enjoyable; once left with the baggage handler, your struggles with it are over. No trying to squeeze it (or them!) into overhead compartments, under the seat, or in the often-occupied cabin closets. Plus, no schlepping it around the airport while you wait for your flight.

Of course, there are downsides to checking luggage, including that you'll have to wait to retrieve it at the baggage-claim area—a consideration if you need to get somewhere right away after landing.

But the major concern is the possibility that your bags will get routed to Dallas when you're headed to Houston. When this happens, it can be a big headache, as a business associate who was scheduled to speak at a medical conference discovered. When her luggage was lost, she was forced to deliver her speech wearing a flowing pair of palazzo pants and an iridescent tunic—an outfit perfectly suited to an evening out, but not exactly tailored to lend her much credibility among the doctors in the audience. For the record, airlines handle more than 100 million pieces of luggage annually, and lose approximately 1 percent.

Whether you check or not is an entirely personal decision, but making the decision while you're still at the packing stage is wise. That's because you'll want to pack into a carry-on bag all your essentials—things like medications, eyeglasses, toiletries—just in case there's a snafu with your checked luggage. To be on the safe side, you may also want to stash in your carry-on some fresh undies, hosiery, and—if you're traveling in casual clothes—a business-appropriate outfit so you won't have to be making excuses for your dressed-down look or feverishly shopping for new duds before your first appointment.

The Fashion Police

Place a copy of your itinerary inside each bag, in plain sight. Because they'll know where to find you, this increases the odds of airlines returning your bags to you quickly.

Don't Leave Home Without It

Besides traveler's checks, you'll need some other things if you're going to be prepared for the unexpected. Here's a checklist:

- ❏ **Umbrella**—The fold-up styles are convenient to pack and can save you from an unexpected downpour.

- ❏ **Raincoat**—Besides wearing it on wet or cool days, it makes a great substitute for a bathrobe.

- ❏ **Sewing kit**—Some hotels provide them, some don't. And the ones in the gift shop are usually outrageously priced. A good kit includes needles and thread, safety pins, small scissors, and basic buttons.

- ❏ **Travel alarm**—Never depend on a wake-up call.

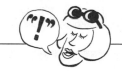

Quote . . . Unquote

In your town, your reputation counts; in another, your clothes do. ... The Talmud

❑ **Clothes brush**—No matter where you are, your clothes need a final sweep to catch any stray lint and smooth the nap.

❑ **Laundry supplies**—Stain remover (accidents happen) and detergent (in case you run out of socks or panties).

Traveling Attire

Consider two scenarios: You're taking an early-morning, one-hour flight from San Francisco to Portland, Oregon, and are proceeding directly to a business appointment. Obviously, you're wearing your working togs. But what about when you're, say, flying cross-country following a business meeting, and are going straight home?

Opinions differ as to how far you should carry the commitment to dress for success when traveling. "Way back when the Pan Am Clipper flew, you absolutely had to wear a suit. And even with today's more casual mode of dressing, when traveling, you don't want to look like a slob," notes one itinerant businessman. "But if you're on a six-hour flight, why wear a suit when a pair of khakis and a polo shirt look very presentable? Even if you are going straight to a meeting, how good is your suit going to look if you've been sitting on a plane for six hours?"

Health and fitness experts argue that you'll look and feel better when wearing light, nonrestrictive clothing when traveling. "Scrunched in an airplane or car seat for hours on end, you certainly don't need to be wearing a noose-like tie, pantyhose that feel like tourniquets, or not-so-sensible dress shoes," wrote one.

The Fashion Police

Especially if you prefer to carry on your bags, consider buying styles on wheels and with retractable handles. It's much easier, and better for your neck and back, to pull than lift.

Still, there are more than a few business folk who believe that you need to be dressed your best just in case you run into someone that you need to impress. One executive even noted that employees from her company traveling on business are *expected* to dress professionally—whether they're flying coast-to-coast or taking the red-eye. "Our company is very strong on dressing professionally. We feel that *wherever* you are representing the firm, you should be professionally dressed."

Even if your company doesn't have a policy dictating dress codes for business travel, there hardly seems to be any advantage in looking like a slob. One small business owner confessed that she waits until she's sure that the flight isn't going to be "hot" before changing into her khakis and sneakers. Otherwise, "I get out of my business cards and network." These tips can help you bridge the gap between professional and unpresentable:

➤ Do wear garments that have some stretch to them. Today, a lot of businesslike fabrics are blended with just enough spandex to provide some give, yet still look buttoned-up. Knits are very comfortable, as are elastic waistbands.

➤ Don't wear sweat clothes. "I don't care whose name is on the label or how much they cost, they don't look professional," states a senior executive.

➤ Do find a happy medium between your pinstripes and your pajamas, which, unfortunately, some travelers look like they're wearing. In many instances, the clothing worn on casual days should fit the bill.

Fold 'Em

If you prefer not to wear your coat or jacket while traveling (and aren't in first or business class, where an attendant will hang it up), use the following folding technique to keep it from getting soiled or wrinkled. Also, keep an eye out for the inconsiderate souls who think a jacket or coat in the overhead compartment is a fine place upon which to rest their luggage.

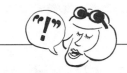

Quote . . . Unquote

The dress coded for business travel at my company is business casual. How much business is in the casual depends on how much time you have until your next meeting once you get off the plane. ...banking executive

A B C

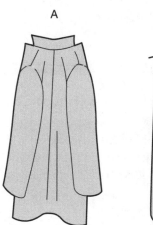 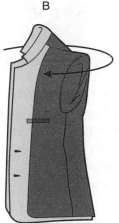 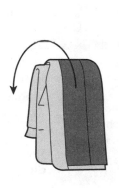

Turn the body of the jacket inside out, and vertically fold in half—taking care to smooth away any wrinkles. Then, fold the jacket horizontally, and lay in a place where it won't be crushed.

195

Upon Arrival

If possible, go straight to your hotel room when you reach your destination. The sooner you unpack, the less time your clothes have to wrinkle. If, despite your best efforts, they have anyway, don't despair; particularly if they're made of wool or a wool blend, you won't be spending your first evening slaving over a hot iron or steamer. Simply fill the bathtub with hot water and hang garments in the bathroom with the door closed. Within half an hour or so, the steam should smooth out most wrinkles. Cotton, silk, and linen garments—which are too absorbent to be steamed—will need to be touched up with an iron. You can also try Charlie Chaplin's method of pressing pants: He placed them between the mattress and box springs overnight. (I make no promises.)

Fashion Footnote

Because the difference between making and missing connections can be mere minutes, low heels are more practical for women who often find themselves practically flying through airport terminals.

On Foreign Soil

Packing for business travel outside of the United States can be tricky: Not only does each country have cultural differences that impact how you dress, the climate also has to be considered. (For instance, in many South American countries, temperatures vary with elevation, not season, and certain areas are hot year-round.)

Fashion Footnote

Will dressing first-rate get you bumped up to first class? "If an airline has an overbooked flight and can accommodate more passengers by moving a couple of coach people up to first class, they look you over before giving you the nod. It happens all the time," notes one well-dressed business traveler who regularly upgrades.

So as not to commit some major fashion faux pax, ask your traveling companions or those with whom you'll be conducting business what attire is considered acceptable. There are also some guidebooks to foreign countries written with the business traveler in mind.

To help you get a handle on the business dress codes of various countries, here are some general tips to guide you.

Africa

➤ You won't err by dressing conservatively. Especially in traditional rural and Muslim areas, dress should be modest.

➤ Business dress is more formal in English-speaking countries, with men wearing jackets and ties. French-speaking countries tend to be less formal, especially during hot weather.

➤ Never wear a safari suit for business; many Africans find them offensive and reminiscent of colonialism.

➤ Even in poor villages, clean, well-pressed clothing is perceived as a sign of respect.

➤ Buildings in which business is conducted may or may not be air-conditioned.

Australia and New Zealand

➤ Seasons "down under" are the reverse of North America and Europe, so it's hot in December and cold in July and August. Dress accordingly.

➤ Business dress is described as "smart casual." "It's like Oregon and Washington," reports a former resident.

➤ In summer, dress is visibly relaxed.

Bahamas

➤ Because of the hot weather, business attire is somewhat casual; lightweight materials are worn year-round, and many business people forgo jackets. Still, you should wear a light suit for a first meeting.

Britain

➤ Americans and their British counterparts dress similarly for business.

➤ The damp climate, and oftentimes poor heating and air-conditioning, make dressing in layers very common.

Hong Kong

➤ Men conduct business wearing lightweight, Western-style suits and ties. (Bankers wear pinstripes.) Women's clothing is generally conservative in style and color.

Israel

➤ In the past two decades, business dress has become more formal—with suits being the norm for both men and women. The biblical-style sandals that used to be customary on businessmen and women are seen less frequently in major cities; however, women commonly go without hosiery, particularly in summer months, when it can be quite hot, and—near the coast—very humid.

Japan

➤ Japanese dress very well and generally, formally—in dark suits and conservative ties. For women, conservatively styled dresses and suits are de rigueur, as are heels.

Korea

➤ Koreans dress very formally and soberly in Western-style clothing.

➤ Businesswomen should wear suits with skirts or dresses—no pants. Modest dress is in order; nothing tight, short, or revealing should be worn. Sitting on the floor is common, so avoid straight, tight skirts.

Mexico

➤ In Mexico City, the business hub of the country, a dark suit, tie, and black shoes constitutes business dress for men. For women, dresses or suits accented with jewelry, heels, and makeup are in order. Unless a host suggests it, don't remove your jacket or loosen your tie.

➤ In resort areas, suits are taboo. "You will stick out like a sore thumb," notes a travel reporter who attends conferences there. For men, stick with short-sleeved, collared shirts and a nice pair of slacks. Women can wear short-sleeved suits (even a shorts suit), colorful dresses, or pants and a blouse in linen or cotton.

The Philippines

➤ Filipinos are reportedly some of the smartest dressers in Asia, so dress more formally (especially for a first business meeting), unless you're specifically told to dress casually. Skirts or dresses are more appropriate than pants for women.

Russia

➤ Depending on whom you're doing business with, they may be smartly dressed or outfitted in flashy, ostentatious clothing.

Fashion Footnote

Pack very carefully when traveling to foreign countries. If you forget something, replacing the item could be difficult, since clothes are frequently sized to fit the smaller and shorter native men and women.

➤ Russian businesswomen often dress in an overtly feminine style; women in masculine-styled clothing aren't well regarded.

➤ Dress according to your status in Russia, where you'll be less well-thought-of if you don't.

➤ It's perfectly acceptable for Russians to wear the same outfit several days in a row.

➤ Summers are very hot, and winters are very cold, but because heating is frequently inefficient and air-conditioning nonexistent, dressing in layers is advised.

South America

➤ Generally, you'll need the same business attire you'd wear in the United States and Europe.

➤ As a rule of thumb, dress more conservatively in countries on the west coast than those on the east.

Spain

➤ Spanish men and women are fashion conscious and will be well-turned out during office hours—usually in smart, well-tailored suits.

➤ Only in tourist or coastal areas will you find total informality in office wear.

Taiwan

➤ Suits and ties are the norm for men, though jackets are often removed during meetings. Women dress conservatively in dresses or separates.

Thailand

➤ Senior male executives wear lightweight suits to work; lower-level employees often go without a jacket and tie.

➤ Thai women are very smart dressers, often donning designer clothes—though never anything revealing.

Vietnam

➤ For initial meetings with senior government officials, conservative, lightweight suits and ties are required for men. Otherwise, jackets needn't be worn. For women, conservative dresses or business-like blouses and pants are in order.

Fashion Footnote

If you have an American Express card, you can call 800-554-2639 (or 202-783-7474) to obtain a weather report and three-day forecast for just about anywhere in the world. The same information for 900 cities can be had by 900-WEATHER.

The Least You Need to Know

➤ Think of your luggage as you would any other accessory—as an extension of your professional persona.

➤ A garment bag or a "suiter" pullman are both ideal when business travel necessitates bringing suits.

➤ A successful business trip begins with wardrobe planning based on your itinerary.

➤ Careful packing enables clothing to arrive without looking rumpled and wrinkled.

➤ How you dress while traveling for business should reflect your professional attitude.

➤ When traveling beyond U.S. borders, you'll make the best impression—and feel less like a foreigner—when you dress in a fashion appropriate to the country you're visiting.

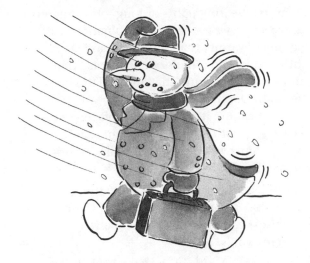

Chapter 16

The Weather Outside Is Frightful

In This Chapter

➤ Dressing for the big chill

➤ Coat check

➤ Right for rain

➤ Under-the-weather accessories

Weather conditions can sometimes turn ugly; snow, rain, below-freezing temperatures, and gale-force winds are all considered normal in certain parts of the country, sometimes for as much as half the year. Unfortunately, when you're a professional, foul weather doesn't give you license to throw decorum to the wind and dress any old way—for example, to pair a sporty slicker or ski parka with a business suit, tote a Daffy Duck umbrella, bundle up in a coat that doubles as a sleeping bag, or don a hat that a North Pole elf would envy.

Don't worry, the alternative isn't to shiver or get soaked during your morning commute. Fact is, it doesn't take much to stay toasty warm (or dry as a bone) when a cold front (or rain storm) rolls in. In this chapter, you'll find out how to look sharp, no matter what the forecast.

Cold-Weather Survival

How to stay warm when the mercury falls? Don't just rely on your coat. Often, what you're wearing under that coat can be more important. Consider the following climate-control tips:

Dollars & Sense

To make a less-expensive coat look less so, replace the plastic belt and cuff buckles with leather ones.

➤ Dress in layers. Wearing tights or long johns under pants, and a shirt-sweater-jacket combination will keep you much warmer than just pants and socks and a shirt and jacket. (That's because layers trap warm air near the body and that air insulates you from the cold.) Don't worry about overheating: When things heat up, it's easy to peel off the sweater or the jacket—or both. The other advantage of layering: It permits you to wear less bulky, multi-seasonal, medium-weight fabrics.

➤ Wear silk undergarments. Though quite thin (no extra bulk!), they're very warm. Plus, a silk T-shirt, slip, or camisole can provide a barrier between your skin and itchy wools.

➤ Choose closely fitted sleeves (for example, ribbed cuffs on sweaters), which keep out the cold better than those that are cut straight and loose.

➤ For women, opaque hosiery provides more warmth than regular sheers. Also, pants are warmer than skirts, and longer skirts are warmer than shorter styles.

➤ Switch to warmer fabrics, like flannel and tweed. Garments with linings will help hold in heat.

The Coat Closet

For most traditional business settings, you'll need a long coat—what men call an overcoat. But even if you don't wear a jacket and tie to work, a long coat is good to have on hand for times when you do dress more formally. Since it's probably the most expensive clothing purchase you'll make, make it a wise one. Here are some guidelines to consider.

➤ While a coat should be roomy enough to wear comfortably over winter-weight jacket, it should also be fitted enough to provide an attractive silhouette—and to keep you from looking like you're wearing a sack. When buying a coat, be sure to wear the same type of clothing that you will normally wear underneath it.

➤ A man's coat should cover his knees; otherwise, it will look too short. A woman's coat should be long enough to cover her longest skirt.

➤ Make sure you can walk easily in the coat. Back vents help ensure that you can.

➤ Buckled or otherwise adjustable cuffs are ideal for keeping out the cold.

➤ Ladies, when considering a coat style, factor in your commute—do you commute by car? Shorter coats, even a three-quarter length one that hits at the knee, will be more comfortable for those who sit behind the wheel— or in the passenger seat—of a car. If you walk or take the bus (and therefore probably have to wait at an outside bus stop), you may appreciate the extra insulation of a mid-calf-length coat.

➤ Finally, buy something you won't get sick of; you might be wearing it every day for four— or more—straight months a year, perhaps for many years.

Fashion Footnote

Generally speaking, your coat size should be the same as your suit or jacket size. The fact that the coat is normally worn over a jacket or suit usually has been taken into consideration in its design. Still, to be safe, when shopping, wear the bulkiest outfit you'll ever wear underneath your coat to be sure it fits.

Coats with Class

The style of coat that you choose deserves some careful consideration, since you're likely to be wearing it for many years. Your best bet is a classic style that's devoid of superfluous details, such as nonfunctional seams and insets, and wide, puffy sleeves; in fact, the less ornamentation the better. If you need to gussy up a coat, wear a great-looking scarf. The following are all good options that have stood the test of time.

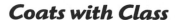

➤ **Balmacaan**—A loose-fitting coat noted for its raglan sleeves, small collar, and button front. Frequently made of nubby tweed or smooth, worsted wool. It's named for an estate near Inverness, Scotland.

➤ **Chesterfield**—A semifitted, straight-cut coat in a single or double-breasted style, usually with a black velvet collar. Introduced in the 1940's as a man's coat by the fourth Earl of Chesterfield, it fits much like an elongated blazer.

➤ **Duffel**—A short woolen coat with a hood that hangs straight from the shoulders and fastens with toggles, rather than buttons. It was worn by men in the British navy during World War II and was adapted as a sport coat for men and women in the 1950's. You'll find it in wool and wool blends and in sporty plaid fabrics. The coat is named for its original fabric, a heavy, napped woolen made in Duffel, Belgium. This style, which is also called a stadium coat, is ideal when paired with casual work clothes.

➤ **Polo**—Double- or single-breasted, the polo coat often comes in camel hair or camel-colored wool. It has a long, slightly fitted cut, patch pockets, and, usually, a half-belt in back.

Dollars & Sense

If you're not desperate for a new winter coat, buy one in January, when they always go on sale and the selection is usually still quite good.

➤ **Reefer**—A takeoff of the British naval coat, it's a double-breasted, semifitted coat with notched lapels and a double row of buttons.

➤ **Tie coat**—Can be single- or double-breasted, with exposed or covered buttons. The latter style, known as a fly-front, has the edge on keeping you warmer because it shields the coat opening from direct contact with the outside.

Coat check: Classic styles like the balmacaan, chesterfield, and polo (left to right) work with suits and sportswear.

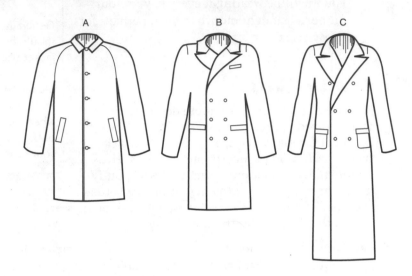

Coats of Many Colors

Especially if you're only going to have one coat that will get lots of wear, a neutral color, such as camel, navy, or black, makes most sense. Choose the hue that best coordinates with your existing winter wardrobe. For instance, if your wardrobe is a sea of blue and gray, black is a better choice than brown. Wild for a pattern? Think twice, unless it's pretty subtle; not only is it difficult to wear patterned clothes with a patterned coat, after a while even the most beautiful plaid may drive you mad!

Fashion Footnote

Even if they have buckles, coats with belts look best tied.

Two other factors to weigh when deciding on a color: Lighter shades show dirt more readily, and darker ones look better with dressier apparel—a consideration if you'll be wearing the coat day and night.

Material Matters

If you can afford only one coat, wool is your best choice—whether it's plain wool, a wool/cashmere blend, camel hair, or tweed. Wool looks elegant when you're dressed up and casual when it's mated with blue jeans.

What doesn't work well for the office (at least for the more traditional places), is a down coat. Though warm and lightweight, it's prone to making you look like the Michelin man or woman—not a very flattering comparison. Save down for the ski slopes, or—in its most elegant incarnation—casual Fridays. Never wear a sporty down coat with a suit.

The Fury Over Fur

It would be an understatement to say that fur clothing has drawn a lot of heat from animal-rights activists. Despite the fact that it's sometimes the warmest coat you can buy (a major consideration in far-northern states in the dead of winter), the idea of slaughtering animals so that you can wear their coat is repugnant to many people—even if they do wear leather shoes and carry leather bags and briefcases.

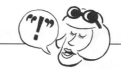

Quote . . . Unquote

My wife Pat doesn't wear mink. She wears a respectable, Republican cloth coat. ...Richard Nixon, Checkers speech

Couple this attitude with the fact that donning fur may make you look as though you're flaunting your wealth or status, and the whole proposition of wearing it becomes a dicey one when you're on the job. As one woman noted, "People tend to make weird judgments about you when you're wrapped in fur. They seem to think that you don't need to work, or won't work as hard." Thus, on balance, from a career standpoint, fur may not be the best choice for a work coat. After all, why wear anything where the risk may outweigh the reward?

The same, however, isn't true for faux fur, which—though it can look rich and elegant—isn't usually mistaken for the real McCoy. Still, to avoid looking as though you're trying to pass one off as the genuine article, save the simulated stuff for trim (around, say, collars or cuffs), and the real "fun" furs (such as those in wild colors or patterns) for the off-hours.

The Fashion Police

What's the difference between winter and summer whites? The cold-weather version tends to be warmer and creamier than the cooler, purer snow-white of summer. However, despite their monikers, neither white is exclusive to a particular time of year—as long as the fabric is seasonally appropriate. For instance, a pure white shirt is seasonless—so long as it's not linen. Similarly, an ivory or cream-colored suit works year-round, provided the fabric is, for example, wool flannel in winter, cotton in summer.

Fashion Footnote

Water-repellent fabric sheds water easily, usually as a result of tight weaves and chemical treatments. Waterproof fabrics, which are usually made of plastic or vinyl, or a fabric impregnated with a resin, are guaranteed not to absorb water. Unlike water-repellent fabrics, waterproof fabrics don't breathe, so they hold in body heat. They're also usually fashioned into sporty coat styles that aren't appropriate for office attire.

Dollars & Sense

To maintain its water resistance, you'll want to renew the repellent finish on a raincoat about every third cleaning—or whenever a light rain soaks in.

A Rainy Day

Into everyone's life a little rain must fall, and chances are good that it's going to pour bucketsful when you have an important meeting—or even worse, a job interview. That's why a bona fide raincoat (and we're talking a grown-up version made of cotton or wool gabardine, not a slicker made of vinyl) is a must for everyone who wears all but the sportiest of work garb. An added bonus for those of you who live in warmer climates: A raincoat can easily stand in on cooler, dry days, and—if it has a zip-out lining—do you right on downright nasty ones to boot.

Gimme Shelter

Raincoats come in nearly all the same styles and colors as regular coats, and the same criteria—neutral color, clean lines—hold true. Some details to demand: a floating back yoke, to keep your back protected, and pockets with flaps, to prevent water from dripping inside them.

If you're lucky enough to have more than one raincoat, women might want to consider not making the second one a neutral color. A cheerier color, like red or iced blue can brighten up a dismal day, and—if carefully chosen—will pair well with much of your neutral clothing.

Into the Trenches

The name alone, trench coat, makes it seem like the perfect raincoat to wear to work—and, indeed, millions do. A long, water-repellent cloth coat made in double-breasted style with epaulets, loose shoulder yoke, slotted pockets, and buckled belt, the trench coat was originally designed for military use in the trenches of World War I.

Aided by Hollywood (especially Clark Gable and Humphrey Bogart, Katharine Hepburn and Marlene Dietrich), it became a classic, all-purpose coat for men and women in the 1940s. No wonder: It's the perfect marriage of form and function, and a superb choice for working men and women, especially when it comes with a removable suede or wool collar and a wool lining. Tan, beige, or khaki are the best colors—considered for some intangible reason to be more professional than black or navy.

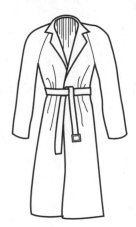

A trench coat provides shelter from the storm.

Inclement-Weather Accouterments

It's not enough to just have the right coat when braving the elements; you also need all the necessary accessories to successfully battle sloppy slush and driving rain.

Umbrella Protection

Fashion Footnote

Those brass loops on the belt of a trench coat actually once had a function: Grenades were hooked to them!

From the Latin word *umbraculum*, meaning "a shady place," the umbrella was originally used as protection against both rain and sun. These days, parasols handle the rays, while umbrellas are used pretty much exclusively to protect against precipitation—to keep you from looking like a drowned rat in front of all your colleagues.

Whether you prefer an umbrella that opens and closes automatically (no fumbling around in a downpour) or one that folds into a compact size (and fits nicely into a handbag or briefcase), the key is sturdiness: An umbrella should hold up when it's gusting, not collapse at the first hint of a breeze. The best clue to quality is the number of spokes: A good umbrella has at least eight, ideally made of solid metal.

Colorwise, you can't go wrong with a solid neutral, but a brighter hue or a handsome plaid is appropriate, too. If you're not the type of person who always forgets his or her umbrella, consider investing a bit more for an old-fashioned, nonretractable kind with a wooden handle—it'll add quite a classy touch to your appearance. Sizewise, pick one that's sufficiently large (a too-small umbrella won't offer adequate protection and can look pretty silly), but save those golf umbrellas—the oversized ones that don't leave room for anyone else on the sidewalk—for the links.

Hand in Glove

Leather gloves, lined with wool or cashmere, are warm and look professional. (The warmest options, mittens and ski gloves, stick out like a sore thumb with a suit and overcoat.) When more casually attired, knitted wool gloves are a good choice. To maximize the warmth potential, buy gloves that don't fit too tightly and don't gape open at the wrists (elasticized cuffs help hold in heat, keep out cold).

Choose a color that coordinates with, or serves as an accent to, your coat—with the latter option being easier for women. For example, until I started reading the newspaper during my commute, I sported a pair of yellow or red gloves that really brightened things up on a cold, winter morning. Now, for practical purposes—that is, to hide the newsprint—I'm wearing black.

Hats Off

If ever there was an accessory that worked better in theory than in practice, it's a hat. Sure, they're a huge help in holding in body heat (much of which escapes through your head); unfortunately, there's not a single style that doesn't leave hair at least somewhat flattened.

Fashion Footnote

A hat, especially one with the brim turned up, creates an illusion of height.

The other, even bigger problem with hats, is that many people just aren't comfortable wearing one. "I feel silly wearing a hat. It just doesn't distinguish me the way it did Humphrey Bogart in *The Maltese Falcon* or Harrison Ford in the Indiana Jones movies," confesses one man. "I'm not comfortable with the extra attention paid to someone wearing a hat," notes a woman. She does have a point; a person is more conspicuous in a hat.

Since President Kennedy opted not to wear a hat on his inauguration day, hat wearing—for men anyway—started becoming less common in the 1960s. Today, the entire practice is entirely optional—for both sexes.

Problem is, there will be days when no matter what the damage to your hairstyle or self-image, it will be too cold not to wear something on your head. On those days—or weeks, or months, depending on where you live—you have several options for not literally freezing your head off.

➤ **Berets**—Ooh la la! Worn correctly, a beret looks great on both men and women. (Don't pull it down on your head; adjust it so that there's some fullness in the top—practice makes perfect.)

➤ **Caps**—The baseball kind in wool can work, especially if you're dressed down. (Understand that I'm not talking about the ones with your favorite sports team's name emblazoned on the front, but rather a solid style without any commercial endorsement.) Ditto those snappy tweed driving caps. But since neither of these caps covers your ears (a particularly vulnerable area to frost bite), a knitted watch cap (or one in ultrawarm Polartec fleece) may serve you best. (For the record, a *watch cap* is the type of head-hugging cap sailors wear.) Just be sure not to wear it pushed back on your head; instead, pull it down onto your forehead.

➤ **Earmuffs**—I personally can't stand to have my ears boxed in, but if you can, earmuffs are an okay option. Just be sure you get them in a grown-up color, lest you look like a grade schooler.

➤ **Hoods**—A better option for women than men, hoods (for instance, the Polartec fleece variety that are advertised in lots of clothes catalogs these days) are very light for the amount of warmth they provide—so hair crushing is kept to a minimum. The fact that they don't fit as snugly as a hat helps in this department as well.

➤ **Scarves**—A silk or wool challis scarf can look chic when tied around a woman's head (think Jackie O. and Grace Kelly). But if you have fine, straight hair (which is usually very silky), scarves tend to slide out of place.

Fashion Footnote

Women, to minimize the ridge-forming, hair-flattening potential of wearing hats, consider lining yours with a silk scarf—a trick that works by creating a buffer between your hat and hair.

Neck Warmers

A soft wool, cashmere, or silk scarf around the neck not only provides warmth but also adds some welcome relief—in the form of color and/or pattern—to what is likely a large, solid block of neutral fabric (otherwise known as your coat). Problem is, many people don't know how to handle the traditional oblong scarf or muffler, and no matter how many times they wrap it around their necks, it still looks like a noose. Here's the drill:

Step 1: Double a long scarf.

Step 2: Wrap it around your neck.

Step 3: Slip both ends through the curve on the opposite end.

Step 4: Position the knot in the opening at your neck, with the ends falling down into your coat.

Fashion Footnote

If you have a coat in a color that's not particularly flattering to your skin tone, wearing a scarf in one that is will instantly perk up your complexion. Refer to Chapter 10, "So Many Options!" for advice on choosing skin-friendly shades.

See Chapter 9, "Accessories: Special Effects," for an illustration of this knot.

Some scarf-buying suggestions:

➤ Don't buy the longest scarf you can find, nor the shortest. It should be long enough to pull off the above maneuver and have about a foot of tail left over on either end.

➤ Do buy a fabric that's smooth, not scratchy. An itchy neck is no fun.

➤ Do choose a scarf in an elegant pattern, or a color that contrasts with your coat (and flatters your skin tone)—say, red on navy or yellow on black.

Foul-Weather Footwear

How you protect your feet from the elements will depend entirely on two things: how serious the challenge (a downpour—or a light sprinkling of rain? snow that's just beginning to fall—or a full-alert winter foul-up?), and what's appropriate for the occasion—be it a board meeting to which you're wearing pinstripes or a day you'll be catching up on paper work and outfitted in 501s.

Because leather is naturally somewhat water-resistant, it can handle some moisture without incurring severe damage. (Suede, however, will stain when wet; consult Chapter 22, "Care and Keeping," for tips on removing resulting blotches.) But that should never be its only protection from precipitation. A water-proof finish should be applied before you even wear a pair of new shoes. Be aware, however, that because these coatings have limited staying power, you'll need to re-treat frequently to maintain water repellency. Worth noting: Leather that's waterproofed in the tanning process is permanent, and a real boon if you live in an area that gets more than its fair share of rain.

Fashion Footnote

If you live in a city where it frequently rains (be it London or Seattle), buy high-quality shoes (cheap leather can't withstand precipitation as well) and rotate them every day; while you can occasionally get by not giving dry leather shoes a day off between wearings, with wet leather shoes you can't.

On days when heavy rain is predicted, but your rubber rain shoes aren't an option, consider a pair of water-proof leather shoes with rubber or crepe soles. Though not as elegant as regular leather dress shoes, they're an acceptable alternative. (Some dressy styles—check out Dexter Shoes' Web site, www.dextershoe.com—are available.) On bad-weather casual days, a waterproof leather chukka boot or duck shoe does the trick.

The shoe story is totally different when we're talking serious slush or mounds of snow—especially if you have outside appointments. For women, stylishly cut, lined rubber boots do exist, as do waterproof leatherlike ones. So chic are some of these boots, they can be worn all day, depending, of course, on your schedule. Also available are rubber overshoes; Totes, for one, makes a pair with the heel cut out so that you can wear them with pumps.

For men, the solution is overshoes, which come in boot and loafer styles. (Totes even makes a slip-on loafer style that looks amazingly like a real shoe!) As for the protocol of taking them off, I'd suggest doing so in the privacy of the men's room (bring a plastic bag in which to place them so you won't have to put them directly into your brief-case). I'll never forget seeing a man removing his overshoes at a reception at The Plaza Hotel in New York City. It seemed so gauche to me!

The Least You Need to Know

➤ When the weather turns wild and woolly, standards for professional dress should still be maintained.

➤ Dressing in layers is the key to staying comfortable when you're commuting in the cold to overheated offices.

➤ A winter coat in a classic style and neutral color looks smart and will serve you well for years.

➤ Trench coats are the most popular style of raincoat for business wear.

➤ The right accessories—lined leather gloves, a sturdy umbrella, a muffler, wool or fleece headgear, rubber-soled and waterproof leather shoes—can buy you warmth and protection and provide the right finish to your professional attire.

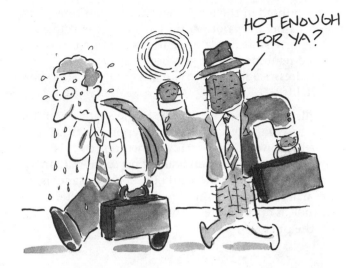

HOT ENOUGH FOR YA?

Chapter 17

The Heat Is On

In This Chapter

➤ Summer standards

➤ How bare do you dare?

➤ Beat–the–heat fabrics

➤ Cool colors

➤ Cool aid

Jobs leave everyone feeling a little hot under the collar on occasion. Such is the reality of deadlines and demanding bosses. Then there are the dog days of summer, the days so torrid that your shirt starts sticking to your back before you're even out the door. That you'll need more than an extra dab of antiperspirant to keep your cool during such scorchers is plain enough.

Problem is, dressing professionally during the summer, when you're alternately freezing in an air-conditioned office and then sweating outdoors, is tricky, especially when coupled with the understandable desire to lighten up your work wardrobe with lightweight, light-colored, body-baring clothes. But how do you dress to keep your cool without sacrificing your corporate look? Just how far can you go? In this chapter, you'll find out how to handle the heat.

A Heat Advisory

If to everything there is a season, summer is certainly the time of year when employees get the most heat about how they dress. "We all just found in our mail boxes a copy of

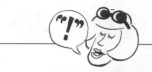

Quote . . . Unquote

What dreadful hot weather we have! It keeps me in a continual state of inelegance. ...Jane Austen

an article printed in the local newspaper about how warmer weather does not permit you to expose yourself more," reported a real estate agent, noting that it was a well-timed reminder. "As it gets hotter and hotter, everyone dresses a little more casually. We needed to be set back a little."

Indeed, just because it's 90 degrees in the shade doesn't mean that a company's standards for appropriate attire are suddenly lowered—especially if the dress code is already pretty casual. "It's an issue of perception. If an employee is sitting in some kind of beach top, sandals, and shorts, a client is going to wonder where his or her mind really is," noted one salesperson, who prescribes a cool attitude as an antidote to the heat. "You can't always expect every little comfort. It's the price you pay for success."

Bare in Mind

Well, it's not always as rigid as all that; accommodations for the weather are made—at least by some companies, some of the time. Since, however, the precise location of the proverbial line that shouldn't be crossed isn't always well marked, you may want to brush up on the appropriateness of donning shorts, sundresses, sleeveless tops, and/or going sans socks or hose *before* succumbing to the temptation. Here, a gauge of what's acceptable.

Arms

Sleeveless is often construed as casual, and even in laid-back offices, may not be correct for women. (It's a definite don't for men, on whom sleeveless garments at work are, quite simply, gross.) The definite exception for women is a sleeveless dress or shell with a matching short- or long-sleeved jacket or cardigan that's worn in public. "I might go sleeveless in my cubicle, but I'll always have a sweater or jacket on hand—even for when I'm just venturing to the ladies room," says one assistant manager. One thing to keep in mind when considering this tact is the condition of your upper arms. Need it be said that only those that are well toned should be put on display?

Feet

Sandals may be the cheapest form of air-conditioning, but in all except the most informal work environments, those that expose a lot of skin—for instance, open-toe, beach or other recreational styles—are decidedly inappropriate. (Wearing them with a pair of socks doesn't help.) Even a fisherman style sandal, which keeps feet pretty covered up, is probably too casual for most offices. For women, a dressy, strappy sandal with a low to moderate heel might work on casual Fridays, or when dressed business casual. What about mules, the summer equivalent of a clog? Usually too casual to pair with a tailored suit, they're best saved for dress-down days—but only if pantyhose aren't a must, since mules look best on bare feet. In all cases, leather is the footwear material of choice.

Legs

According to a 1997 survey by The Gillette Company, 64 percent of working women questioned said their office dress codes permitted them to go to work sans hosiery. The bottom line: If your superiors are going bare legged, there's no reason you should suffer in stockings—unless you have milky-white, veined, hairy, or fat legs. Then it looks ugly.

Shoulders

No matter how informal your office, bare shoulders are never acceptable. If you think you'll want to take off your jacket, stick with tops under them that keep your shoulders covered.

The Fashion Police

Before baring one inch of your feet, consider their condition. Rough, cracked skin and unmanicured toenails should never be put on display.

How to Spell Relief

Even if you can't negotiate a summer dress code that permits short shorts and flip-flops, there are some simple strategies that you can employ to stay calm, cool, and collected—even as the hot-weather gods conspire against you.

High-Fahrenheit Fabrics

Sometimes just shrouding yourself in the right fabric is enough to make it seem as though a cold front has blown in. Surprisingly enough, suits made of wool—albeit a superfine, or tropical variety—can be the most comfortable for summer. These fabrics are soft and fluid, and sometimes gauzy thin, yet perfect for business when woven into gabardine, broadcloth, and crepe. Because the fiber breathes and acts as a natural climate control, it's a good choice for work clothes that will be worn in over-air-conditioned environments and then outside in hot conditions—or vice versa, into the over-heated offices and blustery winds of winter.

Cotton is another natural for summer, whether for shirts, pants, skirts, or suits. The key is to choose garments fashioned of lightweight fabrics—say, a fine broadcloth or crisp poplin instead of heavier oxford cloth or denim. The quintessential summer cotton fabric, seersucker, makes a dandy suit for women (it can look hoaky on businessmen); the most wearable seersuckers have thin, closely spaced stripes in taupe-and-brown or white-and-blue combinations.

Linen is another summer staple, though one that may be off limits in wrinkle-free zones. If, on the other hand, you work in an environment in which linen's inherent tendency to wrinkle is thought to enhance the look of a garment, then by all means, wear it. A plus for linen suits: They're often unlined, making them even cooler.

The Fashion Police

On especially sizzling workdays, anything that has more than a smidgen of polyester, nylon, spandex, or any other synthetic fiber in it is best left in the closet or dresser. Because these fibers trap heat next to your body, they can make matters mighty uncomfortable. (A smidgen, an amount less than 10 percent, is a good thing, since it cuts down on the wrinkling tendencies of natural fibers.) Also potentially too stifling are heavier silks, which will be easily damaged by perspiration as well. Even denim die-hards may want to switch to a lighter weight khaki when it's hot. Though made of a natural fiber, denim's weight can supercede its ability to breathe.

The Fashion Police

Some personal matters to consider when the mercury soars: What material are your skivvies made of? Cotton is a lot cooler than nylon, polyester, or even silk. And ladies, do you really need to wear pantyhose under your pants? Knee-highs or trouser socks should suffice.

Heat-Quenching Hues

Lightening up, colorwise, is a savvy approach to staying cool. In fact, there's even a scientific reason that light-colored clothing is especially apropos for summer: Light waves are converted into heat. What connection does this fact have to the color of clothing? It's simple. Dark colors absorb light (and therefore, heat), while lighter colors reflect light (and therefore, heat).

Fashion Footnote

The heat can amplify a fragrance, so consider switching to a lighter version of your favorite scent or one designed specifically with warmer weather in mind.

Using this principle of physics to your benefit isn't difficult. Even if you wouldn't be comfortable dressed in cream-colored suits (like Mark Twain or Colonel Sanders), a lighter neutral—say, tan, light gray, khaki, even olive—would be an acceptable substitute for the traditional navy blue, charcoal gray, or black. As with your darker neutrals, a colorful shirt or tie could add some zip.

What about white? On women anyway, pure white—whether a suit or dress—is certainly all right in the summer, provided the garment isn't remotely see-through and doesn't look like something you'd wear to a wedding or garden party. (Do, however, think long and hard about whether you want to incur the cleaning bills.) On men, however, it's very *Saturday Night Fever*—which is not an endorsement!

Some patterns are particularly suitable to hot weather. Stripes, for instance, always look crisp, particularly when they're in a contrasting color combination, like black and white. Shirts and jackets "tipped," or bordered around the outside edges in a contrasting color, seem refreshing. What's not appropriate: any overblown tropical prints. Even if based on a predominantly neutral palette, they're too reminiscent of vacation attire.

The Fashion Police

Not only is a deep, dark tan a very passé look, the pursuit of one can lead to the development of skin cancer—making it a practice most employers would probably not find a particularly responsible thing to do. A much safer alternative is using a self-tanning product; such products have advanced by leaps and bounds since the days of Coppertone's QT, and look natural enough to fool even George Hamilton.

Nine Great Heat Busters

Coupled with the knowledge that this, too, shall eventually pass, surviving a heat wave is a matter of adaptation. Some changes to consider:

➤ **Partially lined or unlined jackets**—Linings are usually made of synthetic fibers that don't breathe, making it likely that they—and not the lightweight outer fabrics—make jackets unbearably warm. So if you usually disregard any jacket that's not lined, stop. It's not cheating to wear a jacket without a lining or with an abbreviated one. It's usually not even cheaper; adding nicely finished exposed seams to a garment is costly.

➤ **Short sleeves**—Short-sleeved jackets (especially if they don't require you to wear a shirt underneath) are a real boon for women in warmer weather, but, unfortunately, aren't an option for guys. But what about short-sleeved shirts? While the fashion police absolutely cringe at the notion of men wearing short-sleeved dress shirts (especially with ties), a certain contingent has adopted them—and doesn't give a fig about looking rather geeky. Nevertheless, I still say: If you haven't gotten into the habit of sporting them, you'd be better off not to.

➤ **Shorts**—For women, a pair of the longish, wide dress shorts and a jacket of some sort make a smart business-casual ensemble. The same just isn't the case for men.

➤ **Looser, less structured clothing**—On searing days, you'll definitely want to go with a single-breasted jacket—which can be worn open or closed; double-breasted jackets, which wrap you in two layers of fabric in the front, only look right when worn closed—thus eliminating an escape hatch for heat. For women, a simple sheath or coatdress eliminates the need for constricting waistbands. More comfortable, too, (for women only) are tailored shirts with finished bottoms that don't have to be tucked into pants or skirts. When possible, wear open-collar shirts. Shun turtlenecks.

➤ **Minimal accessories**—Heavy necklaces and bracelets can hold in heat, as can anything made of metal. Likewise, a silk scarf around your neck may eventually start feeling like a wool muffler.

➤ **Off-the-neck hair**—When long hair gets damp and starts clinging to your neck, it can make you look and feel as though it's 10 degrees warmer. For women, pulling hair back into a sleek ponytail at the nape of your neck, or up into a bun or French twist, looks neat and chic. What falls short of the professional mark is trying to put up hair that's too short: If pieces fall out at the neck or sides and a little hairspray won't hold them up, wear your hair down. Try headbands as an alternative to keeping hair out of your face. Guys should step up haircuts, or at least hit the barbershop to clean up the neck area; even if a bushy neck doesn't make *you* feel warmer, it makes everyone else think heat.

➤ **Stay-the-course makeup**—Ladies, the makeup that claims to be long-wearing, smudgeproof, sweatproof, and waterproof really is. Consider switching if yours usually fades, melts, or creases in the heat. Also, instead of loading up on powder to banish shine (which can leave skin looking cakey), try blotting papers, which lift away oil without disturbing your makeup. (Cosmetics companies like Estée Lauder, Shiseido, and Andrea offer them.)

➤ **Common-sense measures**—Carry your jacket (or hang it up in the backseat when traveling) and put it on when you hit the comfort—or get blasted by the chill—of air-conditioning. Men, wear a tie only when you absolutely have to, for instance, if you have a meeting or need to call on somebody. Roll up your long shirtsleeves whenever it's acceptable to do so.

Above all, it helps to maintain a sense of humor when trying to beat the heat. According to one executive in Los Angeles, "When it's really hot and I'm having lunch outside, I say things like, 'Have you seen my jacket?' After the other person nods, I say, 'Good, I'm taking it off now!' And then I do."

The Least You Need to Know

➤ You don't get a vacation from dressing professionally just because the weather turns hot and humid.

➤ Don't let your inhibitions about dressing too casually or provocatively melt with the heat. Shoulders and arms shouldn't be exposed in the office; if done in good taste, legs can be bared and feet somewhat bared in all but the most formal offices.

➤ Wool, cotton, and linen are the coolest fibers; lighter colors reflect light and therefore heat.

➤ Wearing unlined jackets, loosely structured clothing, and few accessories can help you maintain your cool.

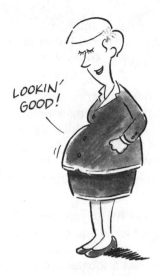

LOOKIN' GOOD!

From Here to Maternity

Congratulations! (Since you're taking the time to read this chapter, I'm assuming you're pregnant.) As you prepare for your promotion to the most important job you'll ever have, you're hopefully happy, healthy, and filled with excitement.

Of course, at the same time (particularly if this is your first baby), you're no doubt a little anxious about the expectation of gaining 25 to 30 pounds and approximately $1^1/_2$ square feet of extra skin over the next nine months. How exactly, you may be wondering, am I going to dress as professionally until D day (that is, delivery day) as I have every other day of my work life? It's a good question, since you're probably going to be looked at now more than at any other time in your life.

The Big Picture

A professionally savvy woman recognizes that how she dresses while pregnant telegraphs important information to her employer, including the message that her job is

Fashion Footnote

Working mothers of the world unite! According to a survey by Playtex, a whopping 75 percent of pregnant women today are employed full- or part-time outside the home.

still a top priority. The all-too-common assumption—that a pregnant woman is no longer up to her job or has relaxed her standards—is still common in today's business world.

Indeed, many working women report that their superiors kept close tabs on their performance during pregnancy—sometimes expecting the worst. Consider Jean's experience: "I didn't miss a day of work, despite having severe morning sickness and gestational diabetes. Several male supervisors made the same telling comment—'I can't believe how well you've done.'"

Unfortunately, not all women ensure that a you-can-count-on-me message gets through loudly and clearly, if at all. "When it comes to dressing, some women throw in the towel very early into their pregnancy," reports an executive at a software company who just returned from her own maternity leave. "While a certain amount of consideration should be given, some women—once in a maternity dress—don't seem to care that they're wearing sandals in the middle of winter because their feet are swollen."

It's not just the clothing you're wearing that determines how seriously you'll be taken on the job. It's the total package. "The accessories you wear with your suit and the makeup that complements it are equally important," explains one manager. Make no doubt about it, this attention to detail will be rewarding both professionally and emotionally. Looking your best is the perfect way to boost your self-confidence, something many pregnant women can sorely use.

Mum's the Word

Precisely when you choose to make your "condition" known to your boss and co-workers is up to you, and in some situations (say, when you're gunning for a promotion or plum assignment), it's probably politically astute to wait as long as possible. In any event, it's certainly considered correct form to hold off until the end of the first trimester, the term during which most miscarriages occur. Many first-time moms-to-be aren't even "showing" by then; they just look as though they've gained some weight. Plus, since they usually still fit into their regular clothes (give or take some adjustments), no one will necessarily even suspect.

If you do need to start adding to your wardrobe while trying to keep the news under wraps, the common wisdom is to choose clothing that closely resembles what you would normally buy and to introduce the new purchases gradually. Showing up one week with a new outfit every day could generate a whispering campaign!

The Fashion Police

The second (third, fourth, and so on) time around, your pregnancy will become obvious much earlier than your first did. With rare exception, these expectant mothers will "pop," or look noticeably pregnant well before the third month, so don't try and delude yourself into thinking that no one notices. It's much more professional to wear clothes that fit your changing physique throughout your pregnancy than to try to hide your news.

The Waistline Is the First to Go

It doesn't take long for your developing baby to make his or her presence known to you. Even though the rest of the world may be oblivious to your pregnancy, your regular clothes will begin serving as constant reminders to you as early as the first month. Waistbands become snugger and—as your bust size increases—you begin "filling out" your shirts, sweaters, and jackets. Fear not, though; thanks to some minor expansion techniques and adjustments in how clothing is worn, your wardrobe can become instantly more comfortable and offer a lot more mileage. Here are some tips.

Pants and Skirts

Can't close that waistband button? Buy yourself a few more inches by hooking a piece of elastic through the buttonhole and then around the button.

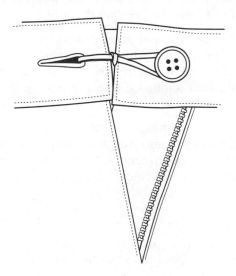

Moms-to-be can breathe a little easier by using an elastic band to expand a waistband.

Please note: By the time you need this little trick, you probably shouldn't be tucking in your shirts—unless you don't plan on unbuttoning or removing your jacket the entire day! According to one working mom, it can be utterly embarrassing—especially if you're trying to keep a pregnancy under wraps—when the button on your jacket pops and a stretched-to-the-breaking-point waistband becomes visible.

Another idea: Replace the zippers on pants and skirts with maternity panels, which are available at sewing stores for a couple of dollars. This, of course, requires that shirts and sweaters be worn over pants and shirts.

Jackets

Wearing single-breasted jackets unbuttoned will give you more growing room, and few minor alterations to a double-breasted jacket will too. Here's how to alter one: Move both sets of buttons to the jacket's inside edges, repositioning one set so as to camouflage the buttonholes. Loop ribbon or elastic around the buttons to close the jacket or simply wear it open, with a blouse or sweater underneath.

Shirts

Early on, wear your straight-hem shirts untucked. (Sorry! This strategy creates a sloppy effect when tried with tops that have shirt-tail hems.) As your tummy expands, make shirts and blouses roomier by opening up the side seams 4 or 5 inches. Sew ribbons to the shirt to hold the sides together, or just leave the seams open. When worn under an unstructured or loose-fitting jacket, no one will be the wiser

"I've Got Nothing to Wear"

Before the day dawns that you really mean these words when you say (or scream) them, you should start planning your maternity work wardrobe. (Prepare yourself for this moment: It can be scary when even your "fat" clothes don't fit.)

It's impossible to predict when you'll reach this point; some women need to buy maternity clothes as early as their second month, while others attempt to get by with larger regular clothes from beginning to end. If you decide to adopt the latter strategy, be forewarned: It can be extremely difficult to pull off if you weren't quite slim before getting pregnant. (So far, I know of only one woman, a size 2, who managed the feat.)

By the end of the fourth month, most women have developed bulges and curves that regular clothes simply aren't designed to accommodate. And even if you can squeeze into them, the fit—shorter in the front as the garment accommodates your tummy, progressively longer in the back as your stance become more swayed—is rarely right.

Sizing Up

Though some manufacturers of maternity wear insist that pregnant women do themselves a disservice by buying any larger clothes, it's a good move to buy a few. Here's why: For starters, because you can. For many women, there's something psychologically satisfying about being able to postpone the move into maternity clothes.

A more practical reason is that you'll need something to wear when you return to work after the baby arrives (assuming you plan to), and it's the rare woman who ever wants to don maternity garb after giving birth—much less when making her grand entrance as a new mom. And since the chances are slim that you'll be back to your prepregnancy physique the day you return to work, the larger sizes will get plenty more wear.

Especially good transitional choices:

➤ Skirts and pants with elastic waistbands. (Since they'll probably be too long, you'll want to hem them to the right length.)

➤ Sweaters and jackets without defined waists. Their fuller size offers growing room.

➤ Trapeze or empire-waist dresses.

Fashion Footnote

How do maternity clothes differ from regular clothes? They're cut to fit and flatter your unique shape, which usually includes expanding waists, chests, and hips but more or less unchanged arms, shoulders, and legs. Maternity wear is sized to your prepregnancy size, meaning that if you were an 8 before becoming pregnant, you'll still be an 8.

The key to making regular clothes work is to know when you've crossed the line into looking sloppy—when the clothes fit your tummy and hang everywhere else. From then on, full-fledged maternity clothes become a better option.

The Fashion Police

Are shoulder pads a "do" or a "don't" when you're pregnant? It depends on your particular physique. If you find that the pads create the illusion of a smaller butt and belly, then leave them in or add a pair. But if the extra padding makes your arms and neck look like they belong to a linebacker, by all means remove it if doing so won't destroy the garment.

Maternity Chic (No, It's Not an Oxymoron!)

You've probably already gotten an earful about the miserable state of maternity wear. Oh, the ubiquitous bows, wide collars, fussy details, and exorbitant prices! All of which is true to a point. But many maternity stores and departments also stock a slew of smart suits, separates, and dresses—clothing that looks remarkably similar to what you'd wear when you have more of a waistline. Honestly, you may find yourself asking the salespeople if this blouse or that dress really is maternity!

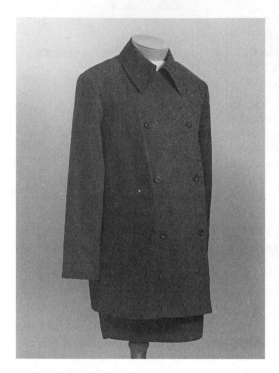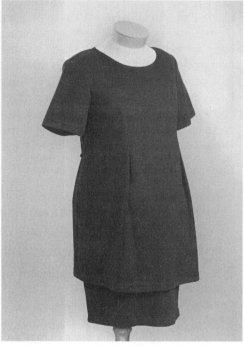

Pregnancy chic. Proof that there's more out there than floral jumpers! (Short-sleeved outfit courtesy of JCPenney; long-sleeved outfit courtesy of Ma Divine Clementine Mom.)

The argument that maternity clothes are pricey can also be made—if you're buying designer-quality stuff. It's certainly possible to find exquisitely styled, fully lined, 100 percent wool suits for $300 or more. But at a nearby store in the same shopping mall, it's also possible to find a fashionable suit in a wool blend for less than half that price.

Some stores that offer stylish stuff at reasonable prices include JCPenney, Sears, Dan Howard (which also has a catalog; call 800-Dan-Howard to request one), Kmart and Motherhood Maternity. More upscale stores—where good sales make beautiful clothing much more affordable—include Mimi Maternity and A Pea in the Pod. The Details Direct Web site (www.detailsdirect.com) offers essentials, including maternity jeans and chinos.

What Works at Work

Whether you're buying larger-sized or maternity clothes, your goal should be to dress as close to normal as possible—it's you, only bigger. After all, why should you suddenly start wearing bows and big collars just because you're pregnant?

It also means no more and no less casual than usual. (According to one human resources director, the biggest mistake pregnant women make is to dress too casually.) No matter what dress code your company has adopted, you should avoid like the plague any garment that leaves you looking cute or precious. That means no ultrafeminine florals, downright clownish costumes, or gestational-gingham jumpers—all of which will undermine your authority in a New York minute.

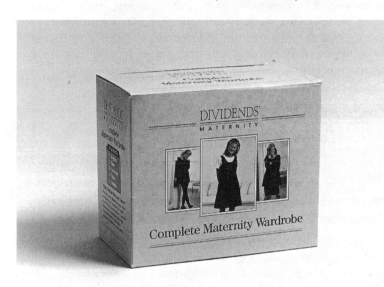

Pregnancy wardrobes in a box, like this one from JCPenney, provide easy-to-wear pieces that mix and match.

The Fashion Police

Several companies, including JCPenney, Mimi Maternity, and Bloomingdale's, have introduced kits (based on Belly Basics' The Pregnancy Survival Kit), which contain the underpinnings of a maternity wardrobe in a box. What you get (though the kits vary) is a cotton-knit tunic, leggings, skirt, and trapeze-style dress in one of several neutral colors. These basics mix and match perfectly, so dressing becomes much less of a hassle. They also work for a myriad of office environments: Pair the tunic and skirt for a city-chic look, or wear the leggings with a crisp white shirt on casual Friday. The kits range in price from about $80 to $150.

The best strategy to adopt is the same one used to outfit the nonpregnant population: Choose a core of basic pieces (jacket, skirt, tunic, jumper, and pants) in a neutral color like navy, black, or gray, that can be worn together or paired with coordinating tops. So you don't look like a plain Jane, buy tops in prints or accent colors.

Exactly how many outfits you'll need depends on how quickly you become bored with the same clothes. If you're more of a clothes horse and can't abide wearing the same things over and over again, plan to have at least 10 completely different outfits at the ready. If you're at the opposite end of the spectrum and wear some version of a uniform already, you'll probably get by with less. Still, the occasional, inexpensive treat can be a well-deserved pick-me-up.

Flattering the Pregnant Figure

What's especially flattering when baby's on board? Some suggestions:

➤ Jackets long enough to hide your expanding middle and—in all likelihood—bottom. Unstructured jackets are particularly wearable during pregnancy.

➤ Straight skirts or tapered pants and sleeves that skim your arms. The idea is to offset your tummy by emphasizing skinnier parts so you don't look big all over!

➤ Showing off shapely legs in a skirt or dress that hits an inch or two above the knee. (Since body parts can undergo rapid expansion during pregnancy, be sure to double-check whether your gams are still up for exposure.)

➤ Creating a long, vertical line by wearing the same dark color head to toe. Or, at the very least, try to wear darker, slimmer colors on bottom—to de-emphasize all that's burgeoning below the waist.

➤ Elongating vertical stripes instead of widening horizontals.

➤ Small patterns and prints, especially on larger body parts. Anything else screams, "Look here!"

➤ Clothing that fits well. Anything too tight will make you—and your co-workers—uncomfortable.

The Fashion Police

Knits are a natural for pregnant women. Because they stretch, they're more comfortable than wovens, which can be binding. However, if your office leans toward the formal, layering a woven garment over a knit—which tends to be clingier—may be the more acceptable way to go.

Go Comfortably into That Long Nine Months

On average, women are pregnant for 280 very long days, making comfort a number-one priority. A maternity bra offers that and more. Designed to expand where you need it to and to provide additional support, these specialized undergarments fit much better than standard fare—allowing the clothing that goes over them, in turn, to look better.

Fashion Footnote

Since knits become de rigueur during pregnancy, the best bra is one with seamless cups.

Maternity pantyhose, which have an expanding tummy panel, are another godsend. (Playtex has even designed its maternity hosiery without the center seam that can be so scratchy to sensitive stomachs.)

Shoes play a big role in how comfortable you'll be, and now is certainly not the time to suffer in high heels. Even if they wanted to, after a few months, pregnant women—whose balance often becomes impaired—can't manage the same swagger they previously enjoyed wearing heels. So, after a certain point that only you can choose, wear lower heels (2 inches or less) exclusively.

If your feet swell (especially early on), bite the bullet and buy a few pairs of bigger shoes. It's a perverse consolation, but sometimes feet don't return to their normal size, so you may just be investing in your footwear future. Best style options: slip-ons, like pumps and loafers, that don't require you to bend over.

Accessories: The Ultimate Wardrobe Extenders

Even if your prepregnancy idea of accessorizing is wearing a watch, by the end of nine months your thinking will probably have changed. Not only do earrings, necklaces, scarves, and the like have the distinction of still fitting years after the baby takes her SAT's, they're inordinately helpful in a pregnant woman's battle to make the same clothes look and feel different—dressy one day, dressed down the next, but always brimming with style. For instance, that slimming but nonetheless plain black dress looks instantly snappy when you wear a brightly colored scarf around your neck. That the scarf also draws the eye up to your face and away from your tummy is a not-so-incidental benefit.

Dollars & Sense

Even if you generally ascribe to Polonius's advice, "Neither a borrower nor a lender be," pregnancy is where you'll want to make an exception. Most mothers are delighted to loan out their maternity clothes. One easy way to keep track of who loaned you what: Identify each donor with a different color of thread and put a few stitches in the label.

229

You can also use accessories to create illusions—for example, a silk "status" scarf and gold-toned jewelry to enrich a bargain-basement suit or a pair of dangling earrings to slim your rounding face. Conversely, the wrong accessories—including belts of any kind and beads that are so long they bounce off your belly as you walk—only serve to emphasize your expanding shape. Similarly, overdoing it with an armload of bracelets or ropes of necklaces can make the big picture too busy. Look closely before heading out the door to be sure you've achieved the desired effect.

The Fashion Police

Lucky you if your legs make it through a pregnancy unscathed—that is, without the development of varicose veins. But if not, you'll definitely want to choose dark, opaque hose to hide the veins that are turning your legs into road maps.

Borrowing from Him

Expanding your wardrobe by borrowing your husband's clothing is one of those ideas that seems to work better in theory than in practice—especially when it comes to dressing for the office. The reason: Quite simply, men's clothes aren't cut for most women's figures, even pregnant women's. (The rare exceptions are slim-to-start women who are the same height as their more thickly middled husbands.) The sleeves and legs of men's garments are usually too long for women, and the hips are often too narrow.

Of course, this doesn't hold true for every garment. But it's one thing to swipe his PJs to wear in the privacy of your bedroom or a cardigan to putter around in on the weekends—and quite another to wear his shirts to work. Even if you could actually get one buttoned around your belly, the sleeves will be more than a bit on the long side and the armholes down around your elbows. The whole idea baffles one human-resources manager, who says, "No matter how you work the clothes, they end up looking sloppy."

Baby, It's Cold Outside!

It would be an understatement to say that no pregnant woman wants to fork over the money to buy a winter coat, probably the single biggest purchase of anyone's wardrobe. But since most pregnancies span at least three seasons, there's a chance you'll need one. If you're lucky, you'll be in your first or second trimester during a very warm winter, plus your regular winter coat will be a style that accommodates your increased girth. But if you're not so fortunate, take comfort in the fact that expecting women tend to be much warmer. Then consider these options:

➤ **A wool cape to drape over business attire and your own coat**—Besides providing enough warmth on its own in milder weather, it can disguise the fact that your regular coat is too tight and even help hold it closed. It's also perfectly wearable for years to come.

➤ **A roomy, nonmaternity coat (think A-line, swing, oversized, or wraparound) in a larger size**—You may need to have the sleeves taken up, but the quality will probably be better than a comparably priced maternity coat. Plus, you can have it altered later to fit your postpregnancy figure.

Beautiful Expectations

As mentioned earlier, looking professional while pregnant doesn't begin and end with how you dress. Physical changes other than those affecting the proportions of your body can also sabotage a professional appearance.

Mane Changes

For starters, because hair and nails often undergo growth spurts, increased attention to manicures, haircuts, and color touch-ups is warranted. Your hair may also become oilier, necessitating a step up in shampooing. Despite the extra time you may be spending in the beauty salon, it's best to resist the temptation to experiment with a new, shorter "do," since:

Dollars & Sense

Need to be dressed to the nines but don't want to drop a fortune for a fancy frock you'll wear only once? Check out consignment stores or your local *Yellow Pages* for maternity rentals.

➤ Most pregnant women look more balanced with longer hair.

➤ Depending on the style, short hair can actually be more work than medium or longer lengths and usually requires frequent trims.

➤ Making such appearance-altering decisions when hormones are raging may not be in your or your hair's best interest. Only take the plunge if you've thought through the long-term implications.

As far as a color change goes, keep in mind that the more rapidly hair grows, the more often roots need to be touched up. If your doctor advises against permanent hair color, ask about semipermanent color or highlights, which when applied carefully, needn't touch the scalp. Should she prohibit hair dyeing of any kind, consider trying the new hair mascaras, which may help blend away any obvious lines of demarcation.

Dermal Disruptions

Pregnancy can have an effect on skin, too, leaving it with more than just a radiant glow. Facial skin tends to be oilier than usual during pregnancy, so it may need to be cleansed more often and/or moisturized with lighter lotions. Two common complexion problems related to pregnancy are melasma—the "mask of pregnancy" that shows up as brown patches on the forehead, nose, cheeks, and upper lips—and acne. Your doctor can recommend a course of treatment, and concealer and/or foundation can help make both less obvious.

The Least You Need to Know

➤ Don't underestimate the value of a professional appearance when you're pregnant.

➤ The perfect maternity wardrobe closely mirrors your regular business attire.

➤ When chosen carefully, your maternity wardrobe can accentuate your assets while drawing attention away from the bigness of your belly.

➤ Accessories can increase the mileage of a maternity wardrobe.

➤ The effect pregnancy has on your hair, skin, and nails often necessitates some changes in your grooming habits.

Part 6
Survival Skills

No, this section isn't a primer to playing office politics, though the issues it addresses may be just as important to your ability to get ahead in your career—for instance, how to wear your makeup and style your hair to reflect a serious mindset (Chapter 19, "Keeping up Appearances"); how you can dress to minimize a figure flaw that's chipping away at your self-confidence (Chapter 20, "Figure Flattery"); how the condition of your wardrobe can further enhance a professional image (Chapter 22, "Care and Keeping"); and how to dress with great style and sophistication on a tenth of what your boss probably spends (Chapter 24, "Investment Dressing on a Budget").

These gems, I assure you, are just the tip of the iceberg of what you'll find in the next seven chapters—all of which will help you implement and maintain your plan to improve your professional profile.

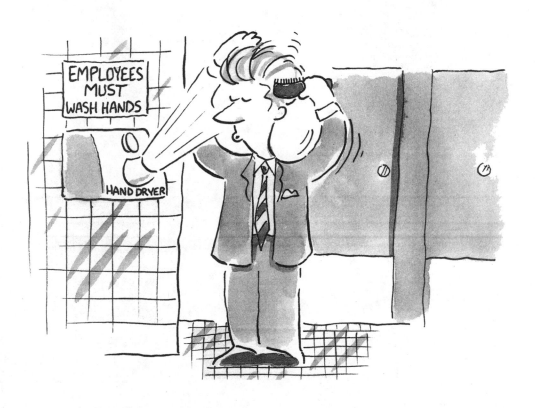

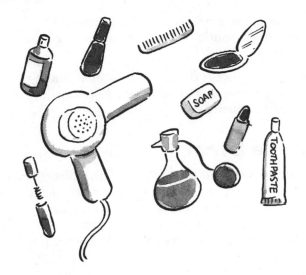

Chapter 19

Keeping Up Appearances

In This Chapter

➤ Tress success

➤ The skinny on skin

➤ The magic of makeup

➤ Beards, brows, and other facial hair

➤ Don't sweat it

➤ A winning hand

➤ Say it with a smile

First, the bad news: Enough studies have been done to confirm the fact that attractive people are viewed as more intelligent and successful, even if they're not. Their good looks often earn them more opportunities than those less blessed in the looks department—including getting the proverbial foot in the door. Like much in life, it's downright unfair.

Now for the good news: How you present yourselves can go a long way toward balancing the scales of injustice, and even tipping them in your favor. But such a feat requires more than just a sharp suit and classy accessories; it demands that the entire package—including your hair, nails, and makeup—be neat and polished. That means that if your hair is three weeks overdue for a trim and your nails haven't been cleaned since you overhauled the engine in your car, you're probably not presenting yourself to your best advantage. Oddly enough, such a lack of attention to grooming seems widespread; it was mentioned frequently by those interviewed for this book. "I can't believe how

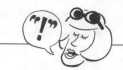

Quote . . . Unquote

What can you do with yourself if all you can do is look good? ...*Broadcast News*

unkempt some people are," exclaimed one manager, noting that poor grooming—just like poor dressing—can be "a real deal killer."

Hence, this chapter details the career boost that comes from being well groomed, and outlines the basics of always looking your best.

The Mane Event

To look the most professional, you'll need a serious hairstyle—one that's neat and finished, but not extreme. Ask your stylist to help you select a style that's appropriate for your hair type, face shape, profession, personality, and lifestyle. This may be a switch for men, most of whom are in the habit of requesting a little off the sides and top, and then hoping for the best—but the reward will be great.

If you're constantly on the go, you'll appreciate a cut that requires minimal fussing, and that doesn't necessitate a trim six weeks to the day of your last appointment. Even better, if you have a facial feature you're not very fond of, say, a prominent nose, weak chin, or protruding ears, a good stylist can cut your hair so that it redirects attention to your emerald blue eyes or sculpted cheekbone.

A hairstyle also should be current (though not necessarily cutting-edge trendy) and in keeping with the image you wish to portray. "I recently made a suggestion to my top sales person that he change his hairstyle, which was slicked back à la Pat Riley, to help tone down his flashy image with female clients," reported one CEO. Similarly, one woman, upon learning that her hairstyle— a French twist—causes her to be perceived as being much more demanding (or, as she bluntly put it, "bitchy") stopped wearing her hair up when in the office.

Re-evaluate your style periodically to be certain it's still flattering, and not just one you've become accustomed to. Even if a cut is your "signature," the occasional modification will keep it contemporary and chic.

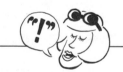

Quote . . . Unquote

Why don't you get a haircut? You look like a chrysanthemum. ...P.G. Wodehouse

For women, shoulder length or shorter (though not severely mannish) is preferable—particularly on older women, who rarely can pull off extremes in hair length. A definite style—even one that's longish and layered— looks more polished than bluntly cut long hair—which is usually reminiscent of high school. Control is key; hair that's too big or seems to have a life of its own can be very distracting. Especially if you're concerned about looking too young, avoid styles that hang down to the middle of the back, pixie cuts, straight-across-the-forehead bangs, and high ponytails.

If you wear hair accessories, stay away from bright-colored scrunchies and hair bows of any size, which can detract from a professional appearance. More polished are hair accessories in tortoiseshell, or brushed silver or gold.

For men, shorter styles are definitely more widely accepted than longer looks—which, rightly or wrongly, are still perceived as a token of rebellion if not out-and-out sloppiness. Unless your hair is curly, it's probably best to have a part, which makes for a more groomed look. To determine which side to part your hair, comb your hair back; it should fall naturally to the correct side. Side-burns, which can help balance a face when cropped to the right length, ideally extend no further than midway down your ears, and are cut evenly across the bottom.

If hair is thinning, allow your stylist to cut it to best effect—which usually means short and layered. A definite don't is to attempt a comb-over to cover bare spots; this tact, sorry to say, only makes the problem more obvious.

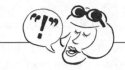

Quote . . . Unquote

You need to give your stylist a true indicator of who you are. When you go into the salon, wear something that's indicative of what you wear to work. Don't go in on a Saturday dressed in some very trendy outfit if you normally wear a tailored suit to the office. ...Kendal Ong, manager of the Vidal Sasson salon in Washington, D.C.

Care and Keeping

In addition to the style, the condition of your hair is also important: dry, brittle, or bleached-out hair communicates poor personal hygiene. Conditioning hair after shampooing will help keep it looking shiny and smooth, as well as protect it from damaging blow dryers and curling irons.

Regular trims also keeps hair looking its best. Hair begins to lose its shape after six weeks; after eight, split ends begin to appear. Regular haircutting eliminates these problems and thus helps prevent bad-hair days. Additionally, because hair that's frizzy or frayed can't reflect light as well as healthy strands, regular cuts also affect the vibrancy of hair color.

With Flying Colors

The many upsides to coloring your hair—the shine, vibrancy, and volume it imparts—can be wiped out if the shade you choose doesn't look natural. "You'll draw stares alright, but not for the reason you want," notes one hair colorist. Most people look best with a reasonable facsimile of their natural hair color, which usually translates into staying within two shades of your natural color.

Part of selecting a shade includes choosing its tone—warm, cool, or neutral. This process is very similar to determining which color of clothing works best on you. Some deciding factors: If you have green, hazel, or golden-brown eyes, you're best suited to shades with the words warm, golden, or red in their names. Pick an ash version of the shade—which doesn't contain any hint of red or gold—if you have dark brown, blue, or gray eyes. Or, go with a neutral shade (like light brown, rather than ash or golden brown) that fall between cool and warm and can be worn by anyone.

Steering clear of a dramatic color change will help reduce the likelihood of noticeable roots—the second worst hair coloring faux pas. Because the necessity for touch-ups can vary from once every 3 weeks to once every 4 months, depending on whether you opt for semipermanent color or highlights, you'll want to know before taking the plunge how much maintenance is involved—so you don't get yourself into a color bind.

A Gray Area

After the novelty of getting your first grays begins to wear off, and more and more gray strands start growing in, you'll probably begin to think about the impact going gray may have on your career. To many, gray connotes just one thing: aging. And in today's youth-oriented society, getting older is not always equated with getting wiser.

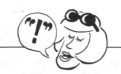

Quote . . . Unquote

You want to be taken seriously, you need serious hair. ...*Working Girl*

Women have known this for years; only a small segment of the female population doesn't do something to minimize the gray. For men, it's a different story: It's only in the last decade that they've—however reluctantly—turned to the bottle in greater numbers.

In fact, four times as many men color their hair now compared to 10 years ago. Another impetus may be the fact that, according to a recent survey from Just For Men, a five-minute hair-color product, men with gray hair are perceived to command significantly lower salaries compared to their non-gray counterparts—a definite drawback if you find yourself in the market for a job!

Whether you choose to cover the gray is, of course, your decision. If you decide to, review your options with a hair stylist before throwing caution to the wind and doing it yourself; because gray hair can be tricky to color, the stylist's advice may make the difference between a natural result and one that's otherwise. And remember, once you start coloring, upkeep is crucial. The rule of thumb: If you notice roots, so will everyone else.

Shake the Flakes

Dandruff is so common that some dermatologists consider it normal. Still, it's hard to have a commanding presence when you're constantly brushing white flakes off your shoulders.

Dandruff becomes noticeable when the skin cells on the scalp—which normally take about a month to form, migrate to the surface, and then fall off—shed at a faster rate and in visible clumps.

Frequent shampooing, which dislodges loose cells, may be enough to control mild dandruff. If not, one of the medicated shampoos sold over the counter should provide relief (sometimes using two or three types in rotation produces the best effect). For those with more stubborn cases (especially if they're accompanied by redness and itching), see a dermatologist; he or she can prescribe a more potent shampoo.

More Than Skin Deep

A clear complexion is a real asset in the professional arena. Men and women who suffer from acne or other skin conditions or who are scarred from adolescent outbreaks frequently are very self-conscious about their skin and have low self-esteem. (They have good reason, too: People sometimes incorrectly associate certain skin problems with improper hygiene, poor eating habits, even alcohol abuse.)

These consequences often spill over into the job: One colleague of mine, a woman who was brilliant at her job and a delight to speak with on the phone, was always very withdrawn whenever we met in person. Until, that is, she underwent laser treatments to even out the scarring that had plagued her since her teens.

The problem doesn't have to be chronic or even very severe to have a negative impact. Even if you experience just the occasional breakout or have some harmless but hard-to-hide squiggles or blotches, you're probably familiar with their ability to severely undermine your confidence.

Fortunately for many, a simple and straightforward skin-care routine (cleansing and moisturizing) is all that's needed to maintain skin health. But, since many skin conditions develop or worsen with age (including adult acne, rosacea, and skin dryness), seeking out the help of a dermatologist if they do may be in your best interest. Dermatologists have a large armamentarium of treatments and medications at their disposal.

Skin Eruptions

It usually happens the day of a job interview or major presentation: A blemish rears its ugly head. The cause? Probably stress, which can stimulate oil-producing glands. What to do? Use products containing witch hazel, benzoyl peroxide, or salicylic acid to dry it out. Taking a nonsteroidal anti-inflammatory (like Advil) may also help reduce the pain and inflammation associated with a burgeoning bump. To keep it under wraps, use an oil-free concealer applied with a tiny brush and blend well. Apply foundation over it.

If the pimple is throbbing or you experience redness and swelling in one or both of your eyes, it's probably infected and needs the attention of a doctor.

Makeup Matters

Forgoing makeup, especially if you look young to start, can make you look unprofessional, less than serious, and too juvenile. Ironically, wearing too much can create the same effects! But how do you strike the perfect balance so you'll look more polished and alert?

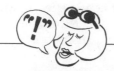

Quote . . . Unquote

I know how to do EBITDA (earning before interest, taxes, depreciation, and amortization). I know how to put an organization together. I even know how to rewire a car. Why do I have to be evaluated by whether I know how to put on lipstick? ...Terry Patterson, the new CEO of Frederick's of Hollywood in *Working Women*

When applying makeup, aim for a natural look that enhances your appearance and doesn't overwhelm. Makeup that looks caked on or is so inartfully applied that all someone sees is two bright pink cheeks and a mouth the color of hot tamales won't help anyone in her mission to be taken more seriously. Soft, neutral shades like warm brown, taupe, coral, or rosy beige are the most wearable and natural.

Think you can't spare the time for makeup? The whole process needn't take more than five minutes, which amounts to nothing when you consider the payoff. You only really need four products: a foundation to even out skin tone and hide under-eye circles (be sure it matches your complexion exactly and apply it sparingly with a sponge to prevent a masklike effect); a blush for a healthy glow (apply it on the apples of your cheeks with a blush brush and then blend well to avoid a striped look); brown or black mascara (a must only if your lashes are very light or sparse); and a brown-based lipstick with a pink, coral, or berry tone to add a hint of color.

The Fashion Police

Unless you're deeply entrenched in an industry that closely follows makeup trends (and approves of employees who wear them), you may be better off saving the colors-of-the-moment for weekends and evenings.

A Clean Shave

Most men are hip to the fact that stubble isn't appropriate on the job—unless they're up for a role in the sequel to *Miami Vice*. But your quest for a clean shave shouldn't leave skin raw, nicked, or burned, either. Minimize trauma as you whisk away the hairs on your face (which total a whopping 30,000) by following these do's and don'ts, which, by the way, are just as applicable to women's legs and underarms.

➤ Don't shave first thing in the morning if you can avoid it. Your skin tends to be a little puffy then, which will reduce the closeness of the shave. Wait at least half an hour or so before shaving.

➤ Do shower before shaving to soften your beard. (When not showering before-hand, say, before a business dinner, first soak your face with hot towels.)

➤ Don't shave using soap and water. The emollients in shaving cream will help the razor glide over skin, thus preventing razor burn. Leave the lather on for a minute before starting to shave.

➤ Do use a razor with a twin blade. The first blade extends the hair; the second cuts it off for a closer, less stubbly shave.

➤ Do shave in the opposite direction of hair growth for the smoothest shave. If skin is sensitive, shave with an electric razor (which causes less trauma) in the direction of hair growth.

➤ Do change blades frequently, or whenever the razor begins to experience drag.

➤ Don't shave aggressively. Using a light touch will spare your skin unnecessary irritation.

If you're prone to razor bumps, a condition caused when coarse, curly hair grows back into the skin, creating a painful inflammation, here are some tips: Shave in one direction with a sharp razor, don't aim for such a close shave (it's better to shave more frequently), and consider using skin products that contain alpha-hydroxy acids—ingredients that help prevent skin from growing over and burying hairs.

Coping with Facial Hair

Some facial hair is just plain unwanted (for instance, sprouting from the nose, ears, and women's upper lip and chin area). In other areas (take the eyebrows), it may simply need some taming and shaping.

Hair in All the Wrong Places

The nose and ears should be hair-free zones, at least as far as anyone else can see. The same is true for a woman's face, not counting her eyebrows. The best methods for removal: Pluck hairs that grow on top of your nose, and very carefully trim those that grow from it (tweezing can lead to infection). To deal with ear hair, consider a battery operated trimmer, which can also be used in the nostrils. Women have several options to hide moustaches and those hairs that crop up on the chin, including tweezing, bleaching, waxing, depilatories, and electrolysis and laser hair removal (the only permanent solutions).

Just Browsing

Everyone, male or female, can usually benefit from some brow grooming, which tidies up a can't-miss area of the face that's often rife with unruliness.

Men tend to have two problems with eyebrows that they find acceptable to fix: the monobrow, when the eyebrows meet across the bridge of the nose, and bushiness.

Both are easily remedied with some strategic tweezing—just enough to create about a ¹/₂-inch separation between brows, and/or to remove the longest, most straggly hairs from the line-up.

For women, eyebrows take on more importance, giving shape and definition to the entire eye area and setting the mood of the face. Severe, straight eyebrows make you look as though you're continually angry, and overly curved brows give you a perpetual look of surprise.

Both can be corrected with some tweezing and makeup. Keep in mind, though, that the ideal brow is generally a more polished version of your natural brow: Change the shape too much, and you'll become a slave to maintaining it.

An easy way to determine where your brow should start is to extend a thin ruler alongside the outside corner of your nose and up past the brow; where the ruler intersects the brow (just over the eye's inner corner) is where your brow should begin. Next, place the ruler diagonally from the outside edge of the nostril, past the outer corner of the eye. Where the ruler meets the brow is where the brow should end. To determine where to create the arch, hold the ruler vertically next to the outside of the iris. The arch should be where the ruler meets the brow.

If getting the shape exactly right makes you nervous, go to a professional for the initial plucking. Either a makeup artist or an aesthetician at a reputable salon can do a good job. After that, you can simply follow the established line. If you decide to go it alone, use a white pencil or concealer to "erase" the hairs that you're considering removing to be sure you've achieved the desired effect before you pick up the tweezers. To "fill in" holes or areas that are too thin, use a soft pencil (and light, featherlike strokes) or brow powder a few shades lighter than your hair, applied with a firm angle brush. To keep brows from looking unkempt, tweeze them regularly. A dab of petroleum jelly will hold eyebrows in place and add a hint of shine.

The Fresh Smell of Success

It's no secret that work can be stressful. But besides the headaches it can cause, stress can trigger perspiration—the breeding and feeding ground for the bacteria that create the pungent smell we know as body odor. The stressed out (and for what it's worth, men perspire more than women) have two courses of action in the battle against BO:

➤ First, bathe daily, and—if your problem is more severe—use a deodorant soap, which reduces the number of bacteria on the skin.

➤ Second, use an antiperspirant, which contains ingredients that control both wetness and odor. (A deodorant alone simply masks any offensive odor with fragrance.)

Unfortunately, no antiperspirant is totally effective (sticks tend to have the most moisture-controlling muscle); even the most powerful only cut wetness by around 40 percent. To maintain protection, you need to keep a reservoir of the active ingredient on the surface of the underarm; it's essential to apply antiperspirant daily—preferably after bathing. (Women can maximize the effectiveness of an antiperspirant or deodorant by regularly shaving underarm hair, which provides an ideal environment for the odor-causing bacteria to live and grow.)

Facing a particularly stressful day? To stay fresh as a daisy (or at least as dry as possible), apply antiperspirant both before going to bed, and then again after your morning shower (or, if you bathe in the evening, apply it after your bath and then again in the morning).

Fashion Footnote

To safeguard clothing from perspiration stains, insert protective underarm shields that absorb moisture.

Good Scents

There's every reason to wear fragrance to work: Studies show that various scents can improve memory, increase energy, even make you less prone to making mistakes. The key is to wear one that's on the light side (a heavy musk, for instance, is cloying and may send the wrong signal) and to use it sparingly so as not to overwhelm your co-workers (some of whom may be allergic to bottled fragrances). If you have any doubt as to whether your fragrance is coming on too strong, ask a co-worker you trust. (And trust me, if you're using one in lieu of a bath, your co-workers may soon rise up in revolt!)

An easy way to safely wear fragrance is to choose a lighter form. For men, an eau de toilette may be a better option than cologne, the most concen-trated form of men's fragrance. Conversely, cologne is a relatively light fragrance form for women and is a good choice for the office. So are sheer voiles and body moisturizers.

Fashion Footnote

If you wear a watch, don't apply fragrance on the inside of your wrist. Since watchbands (especially leather ones) soak up the body's natural odors, spraying your wrists can actually distort the perfume's scent. Better areas to spritz are those that generate heat or produce move-ment, like the bends of elbows, the back, and the hair.

In Good Hands

Before extending your hand in a business situation, take a good hard look at it. Busi-ness professionals need to have hands that are extremely clean and well groomed.

How do your nails look? Are they short and neat, with cuticles pushed back? Men's nails should be trimmed straight across, with about $1/16$ of an inch of white showing.

Women's nails should be shaped in a round oval, with the tips just barely visible when viewed from the back of the hand; extremely long nails that look like weapons are real image destroyers. (If you're into artificial nails, they should look like the real thing: nail art, which never does, is strictly verboten.) Are nails nicely buffed, or—for women only—expertly polished? Hands are constantly seen and therefore, regular manicures, whether done professionally or at home, are important. (A good tip: Chipping is less noticeable with lighter-colored polishes.)

On the same subject, hands that are rough as sandpaper or hardened with calluses need special attention. Regular applications of hand cream should help control dryness, while gently rubbing a pumice stone over water-softened hands can soften calluses.

A Winning Smile

What's the first thing you do when you meet someone new? Smile. When you do, are you dazzling them with your pearly whites or, God forbid, flashing yellow chompers with leftovers from lunch in full view?

Surely, brushing and flossing regularly are not new concepts. But if you're not familiar with all of the modern-day dental miracles, perhaps you should be—especially if your teeth are more of a liability than a personal business asset. Teeth can be capped, bonded, straightened, bleached, or reshaped to look completely natural, often at a manageable cost.

P.S. With regard to the opening question, if you don't like your teeth, and therefore, don't greet acquaintances with a wide grin, a toll is probably already being exacted as to how friendly they perceive you to be.

The Least You Need to Know

➤ Being well groomed is no less important than being appropriately dressed and accessorized.

➤ Hair should be neat, clean, controlled, and styled in a professional manner.

➤ Noticeable roots are a no-no—for males and females alike. If you color your hair, keep touch-ups timely.

➤ Natural-looking makeup will make a woman look more polished.

➤ A man either has facial hair or he doesn't. A day's growth is rarely becoming.

➤ Regular use of an antiperspirant will help keep body odor under control.

➤ For the workplace, a light fragrance in an unconcentrated form is best. A light spritzing will make co-workers happier than a heavy-handed dousing.

➤ Like your face, your hands are always on display. If you're not good at wielding a nail file, seek the services of a professional.

➤ A winning smile is an asset that shouldn't be undervalued.

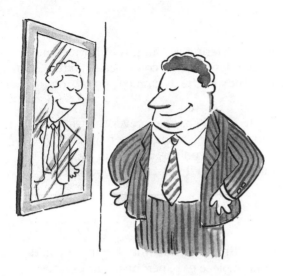

Figure Flattery

First the bad news: Nothing, including diet and exercise, can change the fact that you're 5 feet tall and have short arms and a long waist. Ditto an apple-shaped body and sloping shoulders. Or a barrel chest and thick ankles (well, okay, cosmetic surgery can slim thick ankles and help reproportion other areas, but that's another book).

Now for the good news: You can learn to dress in a way that accents your assets and hides your flaws—feats that have the power to improve your image and simultaneously raise your confidence level several notches!

If you're a man, this notion of strategic dressing might be something of a revelation. Women, I trust, are far more familiar with the concept. Most of us have been attempting to perform liposuction, tummy tucks, and breast reductions on our bodies for years by trying to choose clothing that minimizes this area and enlarges that one. Sometimes we're successful; other times, we end up accentuating the problem.

Well, if you have the few minutes it'll take to get through this chapter, those days should be history. Believe me, once you're armed with the right knowledge, you can meet figure challenges head-on. So let's get to it.

It's Elementary

The first step to figuring out how to choose figure-flattering clothing is to learn some basic principles about the five elements of clothing design: line, color, scale, texture, and proportion. (And I do mean basic, since the study of the dynamics of clothing design is practically a science unto itself.)

If this information is new to you, prepare yourself; it will change forever the way you look at, and choose, clothing, helping you to finally understand why certain garments make you look so great, while others conceal your strong points, and—adding insult to injury—even cause problems in trouble-free zones. As you'll see, it's all about the illusion these elements combine to create.

The Bottom Line on Line

Clothing has two types of lines: outside and inside lines. Outside lines are those you'd create if you traced the shape of the garment onto a piece of paper; inside lines, those based on a garment's construction and ornamentation, include lapels, collars, pleats, tucks, zippers, pockets, belts, plackets, and seams.

Generally speaking, the clothing that's most flattering and comfortable has outside lines that closely resemble the shape of your body. For instance, a woman with a defined waist would look best in a dress that has one, too. On the other hand, choosing a garment that's wide in the middle, like, say, a boxy jacket, could actually hide this coveted asset.

For men, who have far fewer options when it comes to clothing design, this issue is much less complicated. In fact, even the one tricky thing men need to buy, a suit, comes in only three cuts (see Chapter 8, "The Basic Components")—one of which will best compliment a particular physique. For example, if you have the V-shaped torso of Michelangelo's *David,* you probably won't want to hide under an unstructured, boxy jacket.

The Fashion Police

When outside lines taper outward, a figure looks shorter and wider. Outside lines that taper inward make a figure look taller.

Inside lines are either vertical, horizontal, diagonal, or curved:

➤ **Vertical lines** draw the eye up and down, making you appear taller and thinner. A row of buttons, a pinstripe pattern, shoulder-to-hemline seams, suspenders, a striped tie, and pleats are examples of vertical lines. One caveat: When repeated at even intervals, vertical lines can cause the figure to appear both wider and shorter because the eye is alternately drawn from side to side.

➤ **Horizontal lines** move the eye from side to side and emphasize width—especially when two or more lines are used together. Because a horizontal line tends to hold attention (a habit formed by left-to-right, top-to-bottom reading patterns), you'll want one to fall only at a place that you want to accent or enlarge—certainly not a protruding tummy or the widest point of your hips.

Fashion Footnote

One of the most critical outside lines is a strong shoulder line, which enhances all body types.

➤ **Diagonal lines** move the eye along at an angle. They can be very flattering, as they can divert the direction of the eye past a trouble spot without stopping. Depending on its angle and length, a diagonal line can broaden or narrow. Near-vertical diagonals, like those on V-neck garments, lengthen; near-horizontal diagonals widen.

➤ **Curved lines** add roundness. Vertical curves, like princess seams, can lengthen, while horizontal curves widen. A line that curves upward (think of a smile) visually lengthens; a downward curve (a frownlike line) visually shortens.

A

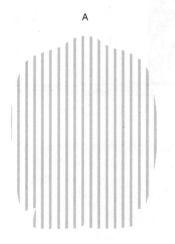

B

Vertical lines, especially when closely spaced, give the illusion of height and slimness; horizontal lines emphasize and broaden.

Color Theory

Color is extremely influential in how the body's proportions are perceived. In general, darker, more subdued and cooler colors (blues, greens, and violets) make the areas they cover appear smaller. Use them to camouflage or minimize body areas. Lighter, brighter, and warmer colors (such as reds, oranges, and yellows), which are the most easily seen, tend to advance and enlarge. Use them to emphasize assets or increase smaller body areas.

Though it's been said before, it bears repeating: A person tends to look tallest and slimmest in an outfit that presents an unbroken line of color. (This unifying strategy also helps minimize individual flaws and a host of proportional problems, including long or short waistedness. The more you break up the body with color, the more noticeable each individual body part becomes.

When pairing nonmatching colors, putting the darker, weightier color below the waist will visually anchor it, as well as make you look slightly taller. Conversely, a lighter color on the bottom will pull the eye downward, shortening you. Worth noting, too, is the fact that color breaks (for instance, when a light-colored shirt meets up with a darker pair of pants) are real attention grabbers—so take care to position them at body areas you wish to emphasize.

Notice how the monochro-matic figure appears tallest, and the dark-topped figure, shortest.

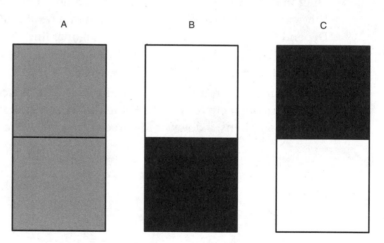

Tip the Scale in Your Favor

Scale refers to the largeness or smallness of design details and patterns in proportion to the size of the overall garment. Though scale is one of the most subtle of the five design elements to pick up on and use effectively, be assured that not striking the right balance between details and patterns can negatively affect the way the body looks.

Things are considered to be in scale when there's not too great a contrast of sizes, something that has a jarring effect. Applied to clothing, this means that small prints, stripes, plaids, and details (such as collars and pockets) suit a petite or smaller-framed figure best, and larger elements a larger figure. You probably instinctually recognized this if you ever said something along the lines of, Oh, I can't carry that off, or I'd look silly in that—with that being a large windowpane plaid or dainty print.

Liberties can, however, be taken with scale to create flattering illusions.

As a general rule, design details that are proportionally smaller—for instance, an itty, bitty collar or skinny belt on a below-the-knee dress—make the body appear larger by contrast; on the other hand, *slightly* larger details—like wide lapels or oversized buttons—make the body look smaller and more slender. Don't automatically dismiss a particular pattern as being too large or small for your figure. For example, a larger plaid or floral will not seem as large in subdued tones and subtle combinations as it would in vivid or contrasting colors.

Fashion Footnote

To see the visual effect of scale, draw two same-size circles. Surround one with smaller dots and the other with slightly larger dots. Notice how the circle surrounded by smaller dots looks larger.

When it comes to picking patterns, it's helpful to know that:

➤ Solids generally make you look smaller than patterns do—patterns can visually weigh you down.

➤ A large-scale, widely spaced pattern emphasizes an area more than a small, subtle, mutely colored print does.

➤ Complex designs or prints work best on simple garments.

➤ Patterns can be used as a tool to balance proportions and direct attention to a specific area, like, say, a skinny upper body.

Textural Considerations

The look and feel of fabrics can create proportional illusions too. Heavily textured, very crisp, or shiny fabrics can visually increase proportions, since they, respectively, literally create more bulk; stand away from the body, thus enlarging it; or reflect light. At the other extreme are smooth, soft, drapey, and matte fabrics, which make a figure look smaller because they, respectively, aren't visually bulky; fall softly over curves; and absorb light.

Keeping Matters in Proportion

Proportion is the relationship of the individual parts of an outfit to one another and to the body wearing them. As a practical matter, by choosing appropriate clothing and/or wearing it a particular way, you can visually lengthen, shorten, widen, or narrow your body and its inherent proportion—which most of us would describe as imperfect.

For instance, because your waist usually falls above the true center of your body, you will usually appear taller, and your legs longer, if you tuck your shirt into your pants.

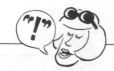

Quote . . . Unquote

There is no excellent beauty that hath not some strangeness in the proportion. ...Francis Bacon

Conversely, you can visually lengthen a proportionally shorter waist by wearing a vest or sweater that skims the top of your hips. Women, who always seem to have more options in these matters than men have, can also opt to wear longer tops to make their legs appear shorter—or vice versa.

A correctly proportioned outfit is pleasing to the eye. While there are no exact rules about proportion ratio, a balanced 50:50 ratio is considered boring. The ancient Greeks considered a body divided one third/two thirds (top/bottom) to be perfectly proportioned—though most uneven ratios, including two to three to five, are interesting. Flipping that formula—that is, wearing long over short—is also a very figure-flattering proportion, particularly for those with heavy torsos.

The Fashion Police

Regardless of body shape, there are a few general proportional tenents that seem to apply to most women. A long jacket or top looks best with a short skirt, and a short jacket or top looks better with a long skirt.

Taller, Shorter, Thinner ... Dressing the Part

By putting the principles you just learned into action, you can become the David Copperfield of dressing, creating by illusion what Mother Nature goofed up on. Here, fashion fixes for 10 of the most common figure concerns.

1. "I'm Too Short"

What works:

➤ Dress in monochromatic or same-tone colors to create a long, unbroken line.

➤ Match your shoes and hosiery to your clothing as best you can.

➤ Choose close-fitting shapes rather than full ones.

➤ Use verticals, such as front plackets, pleats, V necks, and stripes, to create a longer line.

➤ Wear shoes with a higher heel.

➤ Wear shorter (a few inches above the knee) hemlines; A-line skirts, especially knee-length ones, visually cut your lower half in half.

➤ Shop petite departments or at stores geared toward the vertically challenged.

What backfires:

➤ Allowing your top and bottom to carry equal length, inequality between the two creates the illusion of length.

➤ Horizontal details, like trouser cuffs and bold pocket flaps.

➤ High heels; they look out of proportion.

➤ Loud prints that overwhelm; oversized accessories that overpower.

2. "I Want to Look Shorter"

What works:

➤ Create horizontal emphasis with hip pockets, pocket flaps, trouser cuffs, wide lapels, bold belts, and horizontal stripes.

➤ Contrasting colors for top and bottom garments.

➤ Keep the scale of garment details and accessories medium to bold.

➤ Flatter shoes.

➤ Clothing in tall sizes; it's designed to better fit your proportions.

➤ Clothing that fits perfectly. Sleeves or pants that are too short can create an ungainly look.

What backfires:

➤ Clothing styles with too many vertical design lines.

➤ Pants or long sleeves that are too short.

➤ Accessories, design details, or prints that are too small for your body scale.

3. "I'm Heavy"

What works:

➤ Use vertical lines to lengthen and slenderize.

➤ Wear one color head to toe, including shoes and hosiery.

➤ Medium and dark colors, with bright accents near the face to focus attention away from the body.

➤ Strengthen your shoulder line to balance lower-body fullness.

➤ Tapered straight skirts and trousers, which provide a narrower line.

➤ Select longer skirts in soft, drapable fabrics.

➤ Highlight a well-defined waist with a belt.

➤ Showcase legs, if attractive.

➤ Shop for large sizes at regular or specialty stores, where apparel is designed with a larger-sized customer in mind.

➤ Long scarves or jewelry, which reinforce a slimming vertical line.

What backfires:

➤ Billowy, shapeless clothes.

➤ Large patterns and bright colors worn other than as accents.

➤ Pleated or otherwise flouncy skirts.

➤ Double-breasted jackets, which often bunch up.

The Fashion Police

Is your weight holding you back? Chances are that it could be, especially if you're a woman. According to a study by the Harvard School of Public Health, severely obese women have household incomes that are over $6,500 less than those of slimmer women. But even moderately overweight men and women report that the job opportunities available to them are more limited (unglamorous, sometimes unchallenging, behind the scenes posts) than those of average weight—despite superb qualifications. Until weight discrimination becomes a thing of the past, use how you're dressing—in high-quality, superbly fitted, non-frumpy clothing—to gain an advantage.

4. "I'm Too Thin"

What works:

➤ Horizontal details, like stripes, bold belts, flap pockets, and trouser cuffs.

➤ Bulky or highly textured fabrics, like tweeds, flannel, and corduroy.

➤ Layer clothing to create body fullness.

➤ Use gathers and pleats to create the illusion of added body bulk.

➤ Wear brighter or lighter colors, and color contrast top and bottom garments.

What backfires:

➤ Too many vertical design lines.

➤ Clothes that are too tight (exposes thinness) or too baggy.

➤ Clingy fabrics or body-hugging styles.

5. "I Have Narrow/Sloping Shoulders"

What works:

➤ Shoulder pads, extended slightly.

➤ Set-in sleeves.

➤ Lapels and collars that extend horizontally.

➤ Epaulets, a type of shoulder detailing, will broaden the shoulder.

➤ Boatneck sweaters and tees are ideal toppers, since their horizontal lines create the illusion of broader shoulders.

➤ A lighter or brighter color on top to visually maximize the area, or pick skirts and pants with details that draw down the eye—pleats, patterns, bright colors.

➤ Breast pockets add width and detract attention from shoulders.

➤ Standing tall; bad posture exacerbates shoulder shortcomings.

What backfires:

➤ Raglan sleeves, those that start high up on the shoulder (often near the base of the neck), and dolman sleeves, those cut all-in-one with the shoulder.

➤ Disguising shoulders with big collars, which will look disproportionate.

➤ Tight tops, which will only emphasize what you're trying to hide.

6. "I Have a Gut"

What works:

➤ Choose a single-breasted jacket over a double-breasted one—most double-breasted jackets look boxy, and the crossover buttoning attracts attention to your midsection.

➤ Dark, solid colors help make you look slimmer below the waist.

➤ Divert attention to the face with a turtleneck, scarf, or tie.

➤ Accentuate your shoulder line to remove attention from your waist.

➤ Fabrics that skim over, don't cling, to the body.

➤ Wear well-fitting pants—those that are too tight, and as a result ride too low, only exacerbate the problem.

➤ Play up your legs, if they're in good shape.

➤ Long, slim tops in solid colors.

What backfires:

➤ Bright or wild colors and plaids that have too many horizontal lines unless you're covering them with a solid V-neck sweater, which draws attention to your face.

➤ Oversized belt buckles.

➤ Bulkiness, either from pleats or zippers; back and side zippers provide a more streamlined look. Flat-front zippers also provide a more streamlined look. Flat-front (but not tight) or single-pleated pants or skirts, provided the pleats lay flat, are more flattering.

➤ Anything tight across your belly.

➤ Jackets or coats with belts.

➤ Short jackets, coats, shirts, or sweaters; better are garments long enough to sweep the eye right across the middle, not allowing it to linger on your waist.

➤ Very blousy tops or dresses, which can look like maternity clothes on you.

7. "My Butt Is Big"

What works:

➤ Cover it with a long jacket or tunic top.

➤ Focus attention above the waist via brightly colored tops with eye-catching details.

➤ Wear dark, receding colors below the waist, or from head to toe.

➤ Use shoulder pads to balance your proportions.

➤ Select skirts or pants that skim over the hips and taper for a narrower look.

What backfires:

➤ Skirts and pants that cling.

➤ Calling attention to a heavy bottom with a shoulder bag that bounces against your hips. Better to carry a handbag.

➤ Billowy skirts—they'll make your entire lower half look large.

➤ Short, boxy jackets or cropped tops.

➤ Back pockets.

➤ Anything too tight; buy pants to fit your derriere and have the waist altered.

➤ Bulky fabrics, like flannel or tweed.

➤ Pantylines!

8. "I'm Busty"

What works:

➤ Simple, unfussy garments in non-bulky fabrics are the key to minimizing bustiness.

➤ Shift the focus to the face with interesting necklines, scarves, or jewelry; or if you're slender below the waist, lower the focus with skirts in brighter or lighter colors, or patterns.

Fashion Footnote

You are *short waisted* if the distance from your waist to the bottom of your buttocks looks longer than the distance from your waist to your armpits. You are *long waisted* if the opposite is true.

➤ Avoid wide belts that shorten the upper body, thus calling attention to the area. Better are thinner belts toned to your skirt or pants.

➤ Long, fitted, but not snug, jackets or sweaters with narrow lapels in darker colors, paired with bottoms in lighter shades, if your bottom half is svelte.

➤ Woven fabrics or nonclingy knits.

➤ V necklines.

➤ Minimizer bras, which can reduce how large your breasts seem to be by a couple of inches.

What backfires:

➤ Anything tight across the bust.

➤ Breast pockets on shirts or jackets.

➤ Horizontal lines of any kind.

➤ Too short skirts, which emphasize the horizontal and give you a "stuffed" look.

➤ Boxy jackets.

➤ Big collars and wide lapels.

➤ Long necklaces and scarves, which call attention to the area.

9. "I Have a Short Neck"

What works:

➤ An elongating neckline; good choices include V, U, scooped, and square necks.

➤ Shirts open at the neck, to visually elongate. Men should experiment with shirt collars; a long, straight collar may be more flattering.

➤ Longer necklaces and scarves tied below the collarbone will draw the eye down.

➤ Wear hair short or up to give the illusion of a longer neck. Avoid straight, severe hair styles, which can accentuate neck length.

➤ Slender earrings add some length.

➤ Diagonally striped ties can help divert attention away from the neck.

What backfires:

➤ Overcompensating with large shoulder pads, which diminishes the distance between your shoulder line and your neck—thus making it seem even shorter.

➤ Snug-fitting jewel and high necklines, like turtlenecks, mock turtles.

➤ Chokers, dangling earrings, tie pins, and scarves around the neck—all of which draw attention there.

➤ Bulky tie knots; the Windsor and half-Windsor can crowd the neck area.

10. "My Legs Are Heavy"

What works:

➤ Wear darker colors from the waist down, and match hosiery and shoes to skirt and pants.

➤ Choose long jackets that smoothly cover thighs, and long, A-line style skirts.

➤ Divert attention by wearing lighter, brighter colors above the waist.

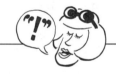

Quote . . . Unquote

He was a tubby little chap who looked as if he had been poured into his clothes and had forgotten when to say "when!" ...P.G. Wodehouse

What backfires:

➤ Straight or narrow skirts.

➤ Short skirts.

➤ Too-tapered pants, which can make you look thigh heavy.

➤ Jackets or tops that end at your saddlebags.

➤ Pants or skirts with bulk-adding pleats and side pockets.

For Women Only: Underneath It All

Depending on the severity of the problem, sometimes all a woman needs to hide a figure flaw is the right undergarment. But when it comes to brassieres, experts say that 85 percent of women wear the wrong bra size.

Do you suspect that you're in this whopping majority? You are if your bra doesn't contain all the breast tissue inside the cup, rides up in the back or front, doesn't provide enough support, or leaves gouges on your shoulders. Make an appointment at a department or lingerie store to be properly measured for a bra. Stores are really pushing this free service these days, and it's a good one to take advantage of.

Once you know your correct size, ask the fitter—who is usually very familiar with all the merchandise—to suggest a brand and style. (If you're over a B cup, consider an underwire bra, which lifts and shapes the breasts and keeps the bustline high.) Even with her expertise, you may still need to spend some time in the fitting room; bras, like all other clothes, don't have a standardized fit. One thing you can count on, however, is that the best bra color is beige. No matter what your skin color, beige works well under the widest range of clothing colors.

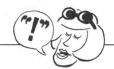

Quote . . . Unquote

If you ever find an outfit that makes you tall and thin, buy it no matter what the cost. ...Lisa McRee, *Good Morning America* anchor in *Vogue*

While you're in the lingerie department, you may also want to check out all the new body shapers. They come in a range of styles—everything from butt lifters to thigh slimmers, waist cinchers, and tummy flatteners. Made of stretchy spandex that usually doesn't leave you feeling too confined, shapers are the answer if you'd feel less self-conscious without any minor bumps, lumps, and jiggling.

The Least You Need to Know

➤ The five elements of clothing design that determine how flattering a garment or an outfit is on you are line, color, texture, scale, and proportion.

➤ Vertical lines elongate and dark colors recede, making them ideal if you want to look taller and slimmer.

➤ Small-scale patterns and smooth, draping fabrics that aren't shiny are good choices when you want to hide problem areas.

➤ The most pleasing proportion to the eye is an unbalanced one—long over short or short over long, not a cut-you-in-half-at-the-waist ratio.

➤ The correct undergarments can make a woman's clothing fit better. The new body shapers, which help slim and smooth, are a real boon for women with minor figure flaws.

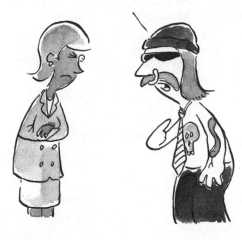

WHAT, I GOT A TIE !

Chapter 21

What They May Not Tell You in the Employee Handbook

In This Chapter

➤ Too short? Too sweet?

➤ Where sexy doesn't sell

➤ The policy on piercing

➤ Ethnic expression

Right off the bat, let's again note that though they're jam-packed with the ins and outs of filing expense reports and filling out time sheets, employee handbooks don't tell you much about how you're expected to dress.

Clearly, part of the reason for the absence of this information is that employers often assume that employees know the sartorial score. "When I was in high school in the late 70s, dress code was part of our typing/secretarial training/shorthand courses. We had to dress up on Wednesday, as part of our class requirement, and we discussed proper dress attire in class. I assumed this was still a part of the curriculum today, but have found that this is not the case," notes one employee, who is responsible for distributing information on dress codes to her co-workers.

The laundry list of inappropriate clothing employees have frequently worn at her office, the world headquarters of a manufacturing company in Iowa, is quite astonishing. Even without benefit of being formally told, you'd assume that most everyone would know that short shorts, low-cut backless minidresses, shorty midriff tops (to show off belly-button rings), and sleeveless miniskirt dresses ("something Goldie Hawn would have worn on *Laugh-In*") are off limits at work.

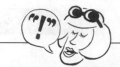

Quote . . . Unquote

Inappropriate attire is like pornography: You know it when you see it. ...political consultant Will Feltus in *Vogue*

Unfortunately, these incidents are not isolated. Employees everywhere are reportedly pushing the limits of good taste and professionalism. "Many men and women in my federal office building look like they're on their way to a workout, or have a date with a vacuum cleaner," observes one manager. Reports an executive assistant: "I work with several women who dress in stirrup pants and too-short shirts that let it all hang out. Their idea of dressing up is to add a pair of gold shoes!"

Many times these infractions are undoubtedly committed unwittingly because the fashion felons simply don't know the rules—especially on some of the touchier aspects of business dress. Other times, the issue is one of taste. Another mitigating factor: As casual dressing has swept the workplace, many of the hard-and-fast rules dictating acceptable attire have been suspended—often without new, clearly defined ones being established to replace them.

If you're new on the job, taking a look at your co-workers and your boss should help you get a handle on what flies, wardrobewise. Try and picture the highest-ranking man or woman in your office wearing the outfit or garment in question. If you can't see either of them wearing it, you shouldn't either. As for some of the sensitive issues, this overview will help prevent you from making any crash-and-burn-clothing moves.

The Long and Short of it

Where to draw the line—the hemline that is. It's a question that women who work have pondered for years. Too too short can be dangerous. ("They can be impossible to work in. Bend down to get a file and it's open season," notes one attorney about short skirts), while too long can be dowdy. (It can, of course, also look perfectly modern, depending on such variables as your figure, the garment's shape and fabric, and how it's being accessorized.)

So, what's the answer? Wearing whatever is the most flattering to your legs, and appropriate for your profession and your desired role in it. Unless you're in a very conservative environment, skirts needn't hover around the knee; an inch or two or three above is perfectly acceptable. Go much higher, though, and you'll risk losing much chance of getting ahead; in some professions, the length of a woman's skirt can actually determine her permanent place in the chain of command. "When you're on a management track, wearing anything short or tight can derail your career. This is the fatal error of some secretaries who frequently dress in shorter, skimpier outfits," says one manager at a financial services provider.

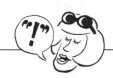

Quote . . . Unquote

Whenever I get depressed, I raise my hemlines. If things don't change, I'm bound to be arrested. ...Ally McBeal

How much leg you show should also depend on how attractive your legs are. If they're not one of your best features, what would you have to gain by exposing them in a mid-thigh-length dress? Even if your gams are great, you need to be sure you're comfortable putting them on display; when clothing makes you feel self-conscious, it can take a toll on your productivity.

Whatever length you're considering, give garments a trial run before buying or wearing them. Skirts and dresses ride up when you sit down (and blow up when the wind gusts), making it entirely possible that you'll be revealing more than you'd expected. On the flip side, some skirt styles (especially longer, flowy ones) can be a problem because they're so likely to get caught in the wheels of your chair.

The Fashion Police

The appropriateness of slit skirts depends on both the length of the skirt and the slit. The safest scenario is a shorter slit on a longer skirt. To be sure, take the sit test: How much higher and more revealing is the slit than when you're standing? If you are, or anyone else might be, uncomfortable with the expanse of leg that shows, save it for an off-hours affair.

Dress Your Age

To look professional, men and women—particularly if they barely look old enough to drive—need to dress like adults. For males, "dressing older" is usually as easy as putting on a serious-looking tie (now's not the time for the one with the bowling-pin pattern), the accessory that instantly provides a certain amount of authority.

Women, however, often trip up here by wearing clothing that exacerbates their youthfulness and makes them look downright girlish—for example, flowing dresses with lace trim, precious prints, Peter Pan collars, or jumpers that resemble school uniforms. "After being referred to as dear for the tenth time, I got the message that I just wasn't being taken seriously," says one young woman who initially wore Little-House-On-The-Prairie-type skirts to her job as a social worker. Especially if you're battling youth discrimination, you'll gain an edge by steering clear of anything — including hairstyles (like flips, pageboys, and high ponytails), headbands, and makeup (anything pink, frosted, or imbued with a scent like raspberry or cherry)—that reads sweet or unsophisticated.

Provocative Is Never Professional

In today's climate of sexual harassment, wearing provocative clothing—that is, anything skimpy, sheer, seductive, stretchy, or that distracts from a message of seriousness, even if it's worn under the guise of being casual—is a losing proposition. "It's frequently offensive to member of both sexes and can do serious damage to your image as a competent professional," explains one headhunter.

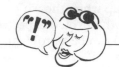

That is a fate from which recovery is virtually impossible. Such was the case with Amy, a mid-level executive at a publishing company, who eventually was fired. "She was a beautiful woman with a knockout body, but she raised a lot of eyebrow. She'd wear all the sexy trends at once, so she'd always be showing off *everything*. Instead of wearing a short skirt with something more covered up on top and a pair of opaque tights, she'd wear it with a low-cut, fitted jacket, sheer stockings, and high-heeled pumps. She looked like a hooker," recalled a former co-worker.

> ### Quote . . . Unquote
>
> You cannot have a career if you look like a hooker. ...etiquette doyenne Letitia Baldrige in *Women's Wear Daily*

That women so frequently cross the line separating professional from provocative isn't surprising when you look at some of the clothing advertised under the guise of being careerwise. One suit spotted in a catalog had a jacket with a cinch-tie waist (tied very tightly in the photograph), and an equally snug skirt that was unbuttoned to about six inches above the model's knee. Its billing as offering boardroom drama was something of an understatement!

But don't think that men aren't guilty of the same gaffes. For example, tight jeans or shirts that too-closely skim chests and biceps—no matter how well they're developed—are too suggestive for the office. Likewise shirts unbuttoned too low are inappropriate—especially when they expose gold chains and hairy chests!

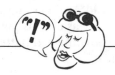

Dressing in a risqué manner won't simply make people uncomfortable in your presence ("who knows where to look?," asked one man), it can also create safety issues. "It's very likely that I could be in a house with man by myself, so I'm very conscious about sending the wrong message about my sexuality," says a real-estate agent. "From a safety point of view, you want to keep an arm's-distance level of professionalism."

> ### Quote . . . Unquote
>
> How did you get into that dress—with a spray gun? ...Bob Hope to Dorothy Lamour in *Road To Rio*

A Tight Squeeze

Wearing clothing that's too fitted and revealing doesn't always mean you're strutting your stuff; sometimes it's simply the end result of some weight gain. Still, just because your excuse is legitimate doesn't mean the ramifications won't be serious. At the very least, because tight clothing looks and is uncomfortable, wearing it can distract you (and often your associates) from the job at hand. Another downside: It practically always makes you look even heavier. If weight loss isn't in your immediate plans, it would be worthwhile to bite the bullet and buy some clothing that fits you properly.

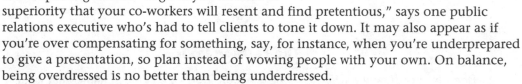

Quote . . . Unquote

I hate to see men overdressed; a man ought to look like he's put together by accident, not added up on purpose. ...Christopher Morley

Best Dressed or Overdressed?

There's no advantage in purposely overdressing for work, pulling out the fine silks when everyone else is sporting cotton. "It gives you an aura of superiority that your co-workers will resent and find pretentious," says one public relations executive who's had to tell clients to tone it down. It may also appear as if you're over compensating for something, say, for instance, when you're underprepared to give a presentation, so plan instead of wowing people with your own. On balance, being overdressed is no better than being underdressed.

What ranks off the charts of acceptability for a 9-to-5 job? Clothing that shimmers or shines; anything with sequins; serious gemstones (other than engagement/wedding rings); low-cut or ankle-strapped shoes; fluffy, feathery or fuzzy garments, particularly sweaters; big hair. Since most everything on this list is better saved for a night out on the town, it's worth noting that when you're planning one, it's safer to bring your finery to the office and change in the restroom—or to choose a work outfit that can be dressed up with heels, jewelry, or a more formal tie for a special evening event.

The Hole Story

Save for a woman's ears, piercing on exposed body parts isn't generally looked upon with favor—unless the pierced party has absolutely no contact with the public. Says one head of human resources, "Self-expression is one thing, but I don't think our company is ready for self-mutilation." Unless you work in a very relaxed environment, tattoos are also taboo. "Piercing and tattoos can easily be interpreted as someone looking for attention," says one executive. "They may be practices that will ultimately come to be accepted, but—especially if you don't have the ability to back them up— they're not the things to do."

Don't Be a Fashion Victim

It's hard to look professional and travel in fashion's fast lane, which will promote the wearing of a skirt over pants one month and perhaps leather with a medieval look the next. Even men aren't immune from fashion's influence: While 30 years ago, Nehru jackets were all the rage, more recently designers pushed suits with skirts and resurrected sharkskin suits. A few years ago, designers were even pushing suits with skirts at men. Fun, yes. Fantastical, certainly. But, as one woman so wisely summed it up, "I live in the real world, not on a runway."

Which is not to say that you shouldn't have a fashion consciousness; dressing in outdated apparel can indicate a resistance to change and a lack of awareness of what's current. The key is to filter the appropriate trends from the inappropriate and then to incorporate the right ones into your wardrobe in a stylish way. For instance, if a wonderfully wearable hue of blue is suddenly all the rage, snap up a shirt in that shade; ditto a new pair of pumps with the hottest heel shape. These new elements will instantly update and energize an outfit, but not make you look as though you're a slave to Seventh Avenue.

The Fashion Police

Don't let trends sway you in the wrong direction. Truly stylish dressers know what styles, lengths, and silhouettes work for them and stay the course.

Beards and Mustaches

In very traditional companies, facial hair—even if it's groomed daily and styled conservatively—is frowned upon. (One lobbyist, who began dealing with the often-conservative finance industry, shaved off a beard he'd had for 20 years on the mere chance that someone could be bothered by it.) That's a shame, since on certain men (say, those with weak or double chins), it serves nicely as camouflage.

That it also is one of the few forms of expression men are permitted isn't completely lost on many in management position. "Men can't change their hairstyle as easily as women, so beards and mustaches are an option they can take advantage of. Long hair is okay, too. We've got ponytails to skinheads," notes an executive at Nike.

If your company seems open to beards and mustaches (and many are, "as long as they're not out of control or worn in any sort of exotic, attention-grabbing style," says one vice president), factor in the upkeep before deciding to grow either. Though they may seem to be fuss free, they're not. Daily maintenance is required to keep a mustache well above your upper lip and a beard

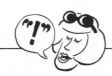

Quote . . . Unquote

It's interesting how people don't reassess themselves very often. They may be neat and attractive, but have teased hair and suits that are so old they're beginning to come back into style. They look stuck, and it often carries over to the way they operate in business. You get answers like, 'we've never done it that way before.' ...Lynn Haneborg, vice president of public relations and marketing, Express Personnel Service from looking scruffy. And, of course, when you're entertaining, between-courses-check for crumbs and flakes is a must.

Is There Room for Ethnic Expression?

Whether wearing a hairstyle or style of clothing that reflects an employee's culture could affect his or her prospects for advancement is hard to say. Thankfully, the tide does seem to be shifting against the tolerance of such discrimination. For instance, after weathering several lawsuits, American Airlines, which had a policy against hair braids (and received some bad publicity as a result), no longer does.

Still, exercise caution: Before venturing into the office in an outfit infused with cultural spirit, observe the tone of your workplace and industry. More conservative businesses voice objection to anything that represents a significant departure from what is generally perceived as the cultural mainstream. On the other hand, those that allow for more creativity and individual expression will likely approve, even appreciate, an element of cultural expression— whether it's an African print tie or vest, a batik skirt, a jacket or dress with kente-cloth trim, or an ankh necklace. Take care, however, not to overdo, especially since African-inspired garb can be bright and noticeable: A head-to-toe ethnic image may be too bold for any business.

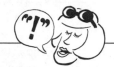

Quote . . . Unquote

Is that a beard, or are you eating a muskrat? ...Dr. Gonzo

Fashion Footnote

When employee and employer don't see eye to eye on dress codes, there can be legal ramifications. Some findings: Employees who are in contact with the public can be held to stricter grooming standards than those who are not. In one case, an arbitrator upheld the suspension of an employee with long hair, stating that an employer may impose a grooming standard if it's designed to protect its image with customers. As for separate grooming standards for men and women, they are permissible as long as they're enforced and administered consistently.

The Least You Need to Know

➤ Though companies often don't explicitly state it in their dress codes, most businesses expect their employees to maintain certain standards.

➤ Though shorter hemlines are allowed in less-traditional environments, provocative clothing, which can undermine your credibility, isn't ever appropriate in work situations.

➤ Many conservative companies aren't very tolerant of employee attempts at self-expression through grooming and clothing. Expect resistance if you challenge the corporate culture.

➤ A rule of thumb: If you wonder whether an outfit is appropriate for the office, you should probably be wearing something else.

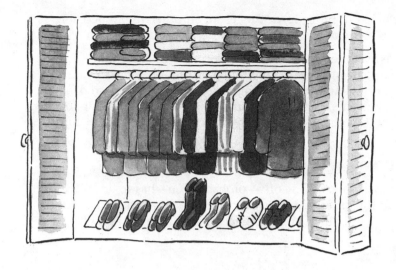

Care and Keeping

To achieve a professional look, you need to know some very practical stuff—like how to sort the laundry and how to store your ties. Because no matter how much you pay for your clothes, there's little doubt that whether you treat them with mindless indifference or tender loving care goes a long way toward determining both how long they will last and what sort of image they will help you project.

Take, for example, a white shirt that's grayed because it was dry cleaned instead of laundered. You don't have to ponder too long to determine that it's going to make you look somewhat scruffy by association—even if you did pay $50 for it. Likewise, a $150 blazer won't win you any points if the lining is hanging out of the back or the entire garment is shiny from improper pressing. And dress shoes with broken-down backs and rundown heels can't help but bring down the rest of an otherwise impeccable appearance—even if you shelled out a king's ransom when you bought them.

The purpose of this chapter is to help you avoid such sorry sartorial scenarios. In it, you'll learn the basics of laundering, pressing, mending, fitting, shining, storing, and otherwise maintaining your work wardrobe so that it looks spanking neat and clean. Think of this chapter as an owner's manual for your clothes, a guide to caring for them so that they last you a good long time—and make you look good the whole while.

Laundry Know-How

Doing laundry may be a dirty job, but someone—probably you—has to do it. Precisely how you do it can make all the difference between clothes that look dazzling white and brightly colored (like the ones in the commercials!), and those that don't.

Sorting Things Out

Sorting laundry is more than just a mindless exercise in putting like with like. It's your last chance to catch and pretreat stains, as well as to tie up any loose ends—like the need to button buttons, zip zippers, fasten hooks and snaps, and empty pockets to prevent snags and tears (and your white handkerchiefs for being washed with your blue jeans). Here's the drill:

➤ Sort by color, separating whites from colors, pastels from darks.

➤ Separate delicate fabrics, which require a gentle cycle, from heavier items. To further protect delicates, wash them in mesh laundry bags.

➤ Divide heavily soiled garments from those that are less so, as soil from one garment can travel to another.

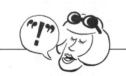

Quote . . . Unquote

Oh wow! Am I being a total laundry spaz? Am I suppose to use one machine for shirts and another for pants. ...Rachel on *Friends*

The Wash Cycle

For best results, the steps leading up to washing need to be followed in a certain order. First, select the wash cycle and water level for the load you're going to be doing. Then measure the detergent and pour it into the machine as it fills. Once filled with water, add your clothes to the machine, taking care not to overload, which not only keeps clothing from getting as clean as possible but also causes fabrics to wrinkle and pill. If adding bleach, do so about five minutes after the wash begins (follow label instructions, especially if using chlorine bleach, which can be tough on fabric).

Hot, Warm, Cold?

Above all, follow the care label on clothing to determine the temperature it should be washed in. (Don't simply disregard the label if its instructions puzzle you—say, for instance, it says to wash a white cotton shirt in cold water; shrinkage may be an issue, or the fabric may also contain another fiber that doesn't hold up well in hot water.) These simple rules are generally followed:

➤ **Hot water** (that which registers between 130°–150°F) is best for whites, items that are colorfast (retain their dyes), heavily soiled clothing, and those with greasy stains. As a rule, the hotter the water, the more efficient your detergent.

➤ **Warm water** (100°–110°F) should be used for permanent press and other 100 percent synthetic fibers, blends of natural and synthetic fibers, and moderately soiled items.

➤ **Cold water** (80°–100°) helps to keep most dyes in dark- or bright-colored clothing from running (provided they are colorfast) and minimizes the shrinking of washable woolens. Cold water is also good for lightly soiled clothing, as well as for items stained with blood, wine, or coffee—any of which may set if washed in hot or warm water.

No matter what temperature the wash water, use cold water to rinse. Not only does it save energy, it prevents wrinkling and makes ironing easier.

Use the table on the following pages to help you decipher the hieroglyphics on your clothing care labels.

The Fashion Police

When washing any fabric that might run while washing, use cold water and wash with similar colors. Be aware that it's normal for dark or bright colors—particularly reds, purples, and blues—to bleed surface dye residues during the first four or five launderings, even if the garments are colorfast. To test the dye's stability, wet a hidden corner of a garment with water and rub a white piece of cloth again the spot.

Table 22.1   Apparel Care Labeling Guide

Icons	Meaning
Machine Wash Cycle	
⊔	Regular/Normal
⊔	Permanent Press/Wrinkle Resistant
⊔	Gentle/Delicate
✋	Hand wash
✖	Do not wash
✖	Do not wring. Hang dry, drip dry or dry flat
Water Temperature	
⁞⁞⁞	Maximum 200°F/95°C
⁚⁚⁚	Maximum 160°F/70°C
⁚⁚	Maximum 140°F/60°C
•••	Maximum 120°F/50°C
••	Maximum 105°F/40°C
•	Maximum 85°F/30°C
Tumble Dry Cycle	
☐	Machine dry
▣	Normal
▣	Permanent Press/Wrinkle Resistant
▣	Gentle/Delicate
✖	Do not tumble dry
Heat Setting	
○	Any heat
⊖	High heat
⊙	Medium heat
⊙	Low heat
●	No heat/air
✖	Do not dry
Special Instructions	
▯	Line dry/hang to dry (hang damp from line or bar and allow to dry)
▥	Drip dry (hang wet on plastic hanger and allow to dry with hand shaping only)
⊟	Dry flat (lay garment on flat surface)
▨	Dry in shade

Icons	Meaning
Bleach Symbols	
△	Any bleach (when needed)
⚠	Only non-chlorine bleach (when needed)
✖	Do not bleach
Iron—Dry or Stream	
⊟	Iron (when needed)
⊟	Iron using High temperature
⊟	Iron using Medium temperature
⊟	Iron using Low temperature
⊠	Do not iron or press with heat
⊜	No steam (iron without using steam)
Dry cleaning—Normal Cycle	
○	Dry clean
Ⓐ	Dry clean using any solvent
Ⓟ	Dry clean using any solvent except trichloroethylene
Ⓕ	Dry clean using petroleum solvent only
⊗	Do not dry clean

Out to Dry

Line drying reduces the wear and tear on clothes as well as the cost of laundering (gas or electricity for the dryer is the major expense). Good candidates for line drying include clothes made of lightweight synthetic fibers and anything that has to be ironed. If machine drying, don't overload (again, a cause of wrinkling) or overdry; clothing that gets bone dry is more prone to static buildup, lint pick up, and wrinkling.

Dry Cleaning Versus Washing

By law, manufacturers must list one care method for clothing, so they often choose the easiest and safest one for them: dry cleaning. That doesn't always mean, however, that the garment can't be washed—either by hand or in the machine.

Fashion Footnote

Despite the name, dry cleaning involves liquid, just one that's waterless. During the dry-cleaning process, a liquid solvent (usually one called perchlorethylene, or "perk") plus detergent pass continuously through the clothes, dissolving dirt and stains, which are captured in a filter. Unlike water, perk won't cause dyes to bleed or run, is unlikely to cause shrinkage, and won't wash out details like pleats.

Dollars & Sense

Wool that you can just toss in the washing machine may sound too good to be true, but the new, specially treated washable wools live up to their promise—thus saving you the cost and hassle of dry cleaning. Just throw them in the machine, wash in cold water with your regular detergent, and dry flat.

What definitely needs to be dry cleaned?

➤ "Tailored" garments—those constructed with facing, linings, and shoulder pads that keep inner construction intact.

➤ All garment made of colored silk, which are often dyed with vegetable dyes that bleed, or wool—unless they're specifically labeled washable.

➤ Also a strong possibility for dry cleaning are garments with delicate or ornate trim, even if the garment itself is constructed of a fabric that's machine washable.

➤ Anything that deserves a professional pressing, although you can always wash it yourself and have the dry cleaner press it.

So, what definitely needs to be dry cleaned? For example, "tailored" garments—those constructed with facings, linings, and shoulder pads that keep inner construction intact. Also a strong possibility for dry cleaning are garments with delicate or ornate trim, even if the garment itself is constructed of a fabric that's machine washable.

It's okay to hand wash and line dry nontailored garments, including blouses, shirts, pants, and sweaters. Some items that definitely shouldn't be dry cleaned are washable cotton shirts, which will age prematurely and probably turn gray when frequently exposed to dry-cleaning solvents. Washing, either by hand or machine, not only gets them cleaner, it extends their lives as well.

Fashion Footnote

Before putting away garments picked up from the dry cleaner, remove any plastic wrapping. Plastic can retain moisture, which can trap fumes and cause discoloring of the fabric.

Block It Out

When the care label on a garment says to dry flat (a common instruction for sweaters and other knits to keep them from shrinking and becoming misshapen), you'll want to block, or reshape, it after washing. You can do this by either drawing an outline of the garment on a piece of paper prior to washing, or by simply eyeballing it. Either way, after washing (and by the way, knits should be dried flat, with water pressed—never wrung—out of them), roll the garment between two towels, pat out gently, and then lay over a dry towel atop a surface that lets air circulate from beneath (racks for this purpose are sold in home-care stores and catalogs). When it's partly dry, arrange the sweater back into shape.

The Dry Cleaner from Heaven

Just as one looks for a good doctor or decorator, word of mouth is the best way to find a dry cleaner. Beyond asking friends, use these criteria:

➤ Membership in a fabricare association, such as the Neighborhood Cleaners Association (NCA). These associations help keep the dry cleaner up-to-date on the latest techniques.

➤ Cleanliness of the store. If a cleaner can't keep the store clean, do you really want to trust him or her to clean your clothes?

➤ Clothing shouldn't have a solvent smell. Such an odor indicates that dry-cleaning solvent is being overused.

➤ Fancy or expensive buttons should be protected with foil during cleaning, as a matter of course.

➤ Jackets, coats, and dressy shirts in fine fabrics should be stuffed with tissue to prevent wrinkling.

➤ The cleaner flags stains and employs a specialist to remove them.

➤ Pick up and delivery are nice extras, even if you pay a small service fee.

The Fashion Police

Never dry clean separately white garments that are part of a set. Depending on how fresh the cleaning solvent is, each component of the suit could end up a slightly different color. This is why Tom Wolfe, the writer who's so fond of white suits, reportedly requests clean solvent before having his suits cleaned.

Out, Damned Spot!

You accidentally mark your pant leg with a pen or spill coffee on your tie. You know you should move fast, before the spot sets, but what exactly should you do? As it is with medicine, the main tenant of spot removal is to first do no harm.

The Fashion Police

Have suits dry cleaned only when they're soiled (for instance, if you've perspired clear through to the lining) or if you'll be packing them away for a season (moths feed off the stains in natural fibers). Otherwise, give a suit a good brushing after each wear to remove any surface dirt and allow it to air out for a few days before wearing again.

Emergency Measures

Whether you're going to try to remove a stain yourself, or plan to turn it over to a pro, there are some measures you should take immediately after being spotted to contain the damage:

➤ Scrape off any loose surface matter and/or blot up all the liquid you can, using a clean cloth, tissue, or paper towel.

Fashion Footnote

Cosmetics, pen ink, and butter are oil-based stains. These characteristically show up as darker patches that are completely absorbed into the material. Wine, vinegar, and coffee are water-based stains, which usually bead up for a few seconds before being absorbed into the fabric; they often dry a little stiff. Some stains, like tomato sauce, coffee with cream, salad dressing, and chocolate, are combination stains.

➤ If you have a greasy or oily spot, dust some talcum powder or cornstarch on it. As the powder absorbs the stain, it will become gummy. Scrape off the powder after a few minutes and continue reapplying and scraping fresh powder until it no longer seems to be absorbing the oil or grease (if you can, leave the powder on overnight). If you're lucky, this method will completely absorb the stain. An alternative is to apply an instant spot remover, which is basically a dry-cleaning solvent. These products can be used on all types of fabrics and don't require any further washing. One over-the-counter brand that professional dry cleaners recommend is Carbona; another is Energine.

➤ If the stain isn't oil based and the item is washable (like most cottons and many synthetics), or is constructed of a smooth silk, rayon, or wool, pour a tablespoon of room-temperature water on the affected area. This effort will help dilute the stain and remove some of it while it's still fresh, thereby minimizing the potential damage.

➤ For best results, take further action within the next day or two. Promptness is key, since the longer a spot sits, the longer oxidation has to do its dirty work, and it's this process that turns a spot into a full-fledged stain.

Don't Try This Trick at Home

A dry cleaner that specializes in spot removal (or a *spotter* in dry-cleaning terminology) may be your best bet when certain stains appear in your lap or on your lapel.

Safer in the cleaner's hands than in yours, for instance, are spots or stains on colored silk, linen, or rayon—fabrics in which it's easy to rub off some dye during the cleaning process and leave a sometimes bigger blemish than the original stain. Also risky to self-treat are spots of unknown origin, since a remedy as common as dabbing with water can cause certain stains—for example, those that are oil based—to coagulate and become more difficult to remove. Finally, on the don't-even-think-about-it list are spots on very expensive garments or those to which you have a strong attachment. If you muck up a rescue attempt on these, you'll never forgive yourself!

Going It Alone

There are scads of do-it-yourself stain removal methods, many of which require you to have at the ready an arsenal of ingredients—which you wouldn't otherwise have on hand. I prefer to use a commercial stain removal product.

Many stains can be effectively handled at home with a product like Spray 'n Wash or Shout. In a test conducted on 16 prewash products by the Good Housekeeping Institute, all 16 performed well on common stains, such as ink, lipstick, coffee, Italian dressing, and wine. One caveat: Be sure a stain is completely removed before drying the garment in the dryer or ironing it; heat will set a stain, making it virtually impossible to remove.

Spotlight on Stain Removers

All stain removers work equally well (according to the Good Housekeeping Institute report) but vary in the way they are used. Only the stick form can be applied up to one week before washing, making it ideal for those who are likely to treat a stain when it's fresh and then forget about washing it the next day. Liquid and aerosol stain removers (which are formulated to dissolve oily stains) should be applied just prior to laundering and not be allowed to

Fashion Footnote

Invisible stains—those that don't show up until a garment is laundered or dry cleaned—are caused by tannins, plant-based substances often found in colorless beverages like alcohol. (They're also in fruit juices and tomato and soy sauce.) Usually undetectable to the naked eye, the heat from dryers or irons speeds up the oxidation process, causing a stain to—not so mysteriously anymore—appear.

dry, to avoid color change or loss. Garments treated with gel stain removers should be washed within an hour.

Pressing Matters

To get around the fear and/or disdain you have for ironing your clothes, you can rely almost totally on a dry cleaner to keep your wardrobe pressed to the nines. But for such services, you will pay dearly, and even then, you'll still inevitably have to do some occasional touching-up. So, while you don't have to become an expert in home economics, it is necessary to know how to wield an iron.

The Fashion Police

Buy a steam iron with a nonstick coating and a clearly visible water-level indicator—the heavier, the better. An ironing board should be well padded and covered in cotton canvas; metallic covers can cause heat to bounce back, damaging delicate fabrics.

The Iron Age

Before getting down to any pressing business, you should do the following:

1. Set the temperature dial on the iron for the fabric you're ironing; this step is crucial, since different fabrics tolerate different amounts of heat. Use the coolest setting that will get the job done.

Fashion Footnote

An ironing board is the right height for you when you can stand with your arms hanging straight down and your hand is flat on the board.

2. Fill the iron with water (distilled water helps prevent mineral build-up in the steam holes but is not as critical as it once was—newer irons are designed to prevent such build-up). No garment should be ironed bone-dry; moisture protects against scorching and other heat-related disasters. Other alternatives to using the steam from the iron: Press clothes when they're damp (either don't dry them all the way or dampen them with water from a spray bottle) or lightly spritz them with spray starch—a method that's most effective on natural fibers and rayon and when you're using a dry iron.

3. Have at the ready a pressing cloth to place between the iron and the fabric on garments that are prone to turning shiny—for instance, anything made of wool or silk. To eliminate this problem, choose an iron with an aluminum sole plate or outfit your iron with a fabric "slipper" sold at sewing-supply stores.

Pressing Pointers

The exact technique you should use to iron a garment is your choice; there are many ways, and—as they say—different strokes for different folks. It's worth noting that many experts recommend first doing the detail and inside work, such as cuffs, waistbands, pockets, and collars, and then finishing with the flat ironing. In any event, pay attention to these do's and don'ts, on which many professionals agree:

➤ Don't iron over any area that's soiled or stained. Heat sets stains.

➤ Do iron on the wrong side of fabrics whenever possible to prevent color fading.

➤ Don't iron hemlines or other folds with a heavy hand; if you do an indentation may form on the right side of the fabric. Use a press cloth or a damp washcloth, to be safe.

➤ Do use small amounts—not large doses—of spray starch, respraying if necessary.

➤ To use the iron most effectively, do work the pointed end into hard-to-reach areas, such as under the sides of a shirt's back pleat.

➤ Don't start ironing a garment in a conspicuous spot, like the front of a shirt. Test the heat of the iron on an inconspicuous area such as the back bottom.

➤ If you're ironing several pieces at one time, iron garments that require a lower heat setting first and then raise the temperature of the iron as needed for other garments. This way you're less likely to accidentally iron pieces at too high a temperature.

Fashion Footnote

Ironing is when you move the iron back and forth over flat areas. *Pressing* is the up-and-down, in-and-out motion used to enhance the basic shape of a garment and to do detail work like sneaking around buttons and smoothing cuffs.

Fashion Footnote

How to know where to press creases on pants? When the inseam and outside seam are placed one on top of the other, the crease should fall on the fold.

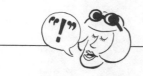

Quote . . . Unquote

Expecting a flood? ...*Yellow Pages'*
advertisement for tailors

Having a Fit

A tailor is like a plastic surgeon for clothing, nipping
and tucking to change what isn't—or never was—right
and to give a lift to those things (like a seasons' old,
oversized jacket) that are showing their age. When you
find a skilled tailor (word-of-mouth is the best way, by
far), he or she should be treasured, because true talent
can transform ill-fitting garments into clothing that
looks custom-made—the hallmark of a successful man
and woman's wardrobe.

Alterations: Minor Adjustments or Major Overhaul?

The simplest, and least expensive, alterations involve basic repairs (such as repositioning a drooping lining) and minor adjustments to the fit of a garment—for example,
taking in side seams and waistbands or shortening hems and sleeves. Length alterations are very common because most people aren't symmetrical; one leg or arm is
often longer than the other, or one hip is higher.

The Fashion Police

A garment can't be all things to all shoes. Pants and skirts should be hemmed to a specific
shoe or heel height. If you try to accommodate both your flats and your heels (or your lug
soles and your finest footwear), the garment simply won't look right with either.

More complicated (and expensive), but by no means impossible to do, are fixes that
help update or change the design of a garment—for instance, reshaping jacket lapels,
adding a slit to a skirt, and narrowing pants that are too wide.

At the farthest end of the difficulty spectrum are changes to the shoulder area, collar,
armhole, or neckline—all of which necessitate other changes. (Even downsizing
shoulder pads can sometimes mean a slew of other adjustments.)

And because of the work and many changes involved, it's usually not worth overhaul-
ing the basic design or proportions of a garment, especially if you're considering
buying the garment new and having it altered. It might make sense to spend the
money on alterations if you already own—and otherwise love—the garment. But
unless it's been markedly reduced, when you factor in the cost of alterations, you're
probably better off looking for another garment that's closer to your ideal.

Reweaving: Who, What, When, Why, and How?

When does it pay to reweave a jacket that has an obvious gash in the fabric or a pair of pants marred by a cigarette burn? Obviously, it's not worth reweaving a garment if it would cost less to replace it with something new, or if it's so worn that a new problem is likely to crop up shortly thereafter. *Reweaving,* a process in which a missing area is painstakingly recreated so that the weave and pattern are duplicated exactly via tiny, precise stitches, usually with threads taken from the marred garment, is really a service that should be saved for your most valuable or beloved garments.

Certain fabrics (including tightly woven ones, as well as the ever-popular work fabric, gabardine) are very difficult to reweave, whereas some fabrics with complicated patterns—such as herringbone and tweeds—are relatively easy. To find out whether a defect can be rewoven, you'll need to track down an expert in this dying art. Your first step: Ask your dry cleaner for a recommendation.

When reweaving—which can easily cost upwards of $50—isn't a viable option, some less-expensive, alternative repair methods are darning and patching.

Dollars & Sense

When faced with the option of either buying a garment that fits your hips and having the waist taken in by a tailor, or doing the opposite, go with the first choice. Having a waistband made smaller is a relatively simple and inexpensive fix compared to altering the hips. Plus, depending on how a garment is constructed, hip alterations may not be possible.

Making A-Mends

Clothes can be high-maintenance items. Luckily, the little chores required to keep clothing in good wearing condition are less annoying when you have some basic knowledge and equipment.

What a Pill!

Pills, those little balls of fibers that break off and cling tenaciously to the surface, can quickly spoil the look of a garment. (Synthetic fibers, like polyester, nylon, and acrylic are especially prone to pilling because they're strong.) Sheer off pills with a razor, pumice stone, a defuzzing gadget, or even scissors (for spot fixes). The stronger the fabric, the firmer your strokes can be; always hold the fabric taut.

No Hint of Lint

The plastic paddle with the velvety surface that's sold in drug stores is ideal for removing lint. Simply brush it lightly over the fabric's surface. (If you find you're just making a big mess, either brush in the opposite direction or turn the brush over and brush in the same direction.) To clean the paddle, wipe along—never across—the ribs. In an emergency, use tape to defuzz.

Smooth a Pull

If a pulled yarn can't be redistributed by stretching the fabric, use a crochet hook to pull the extra yarn to the back of the fabric. Once there, it may eventually work itself back into the fabric. If it doesn't, knot the loop against the back of the fabric or tack it down with a few stitches.

Buttoning Up

It's not surprising that buttons are always popping off. Most buttons on clothing are sewn on by a machine that goes from button to button to button, snipping the thread in between—hardly a secure beginning! To reattach, follow these instructions:

1. Use a piece of thread that's doubled and then knotted at the end.

2. Holding the button in place, send the needle from the back of the fabric up through one of the holes. To keep from sewing the button on too tightly (which causes stress on the fabric and makes it difficult to button), create a thread *shank,* a space between the fabric and the button, by placing a toothpick or a bobby pin across the top of the button. (On a heavy coat, you might have to use a pencil.)

3. Stitch down over the toothpick (working either side to side or crisscross) into the next hole, then up again into the next, until each set of holes has been bound five or six times. (For extra protection on a four-hole button, sew thread through only two holes at a time. This way, should one set break loose, the other side will still hold the button.)

4. Remove the toothpick; lift the button away from the fabric so that the stitches become taut, and wrap the thread around the exposed threads between the button and fabric several times. Make a stitch into the shank to secure it and then tie off the thread under the button.

When sewing on a button, a thread shank allows the button to slip through the buttonhole more easily.

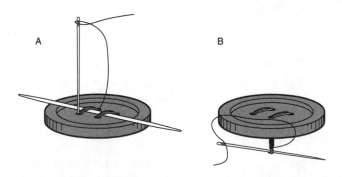

A

B

The Fashion Police

Loose threads on a garment should always be cut. Pulling can cause a chain reaction that allows an entire seam to open up.

Securing a Hem

We ask a lot of hems, considering that they're held up by only one strand of thread! Still, it's rare that an entire hem comes falling down; usually just a small portion—say, the section that gets caught in your heel—comes undone. You can secure a falling hem by using either the uneven slipstitch, which is ideal when the hem's edge is folded, or a blind-hemming stitch, a particularly good stabilizing stitch, since the stitches are taken inside (between the hem and the garment) where they're less exposed to wear and tear.

To keep thread from getting tangled, use a single thread that's only about 18 to 24 inches long. Knot it at one end. To tie off thread after completing your hand stitching, take a tiny stitch behind the last entry point of the thread into the underside of the fabric. Pull your needle and thread through, leaving a small thread loop. Take another short backstitch in the same place, but pass your needle and thread through the loop of the first stitch. Then pull both stitches close to the fabric and cut the thread.

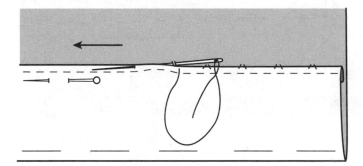

How to sew the uneven slipstitch: Begin by fastening the thread on the wrong side of the hem, bringing your needle and thread through the hem edge. Working from right to left, take a small stitch in the garment, catching only a single yarn. Next, opposite that stitch, insert the needle and slip through the fold for about 1/4 inch. Continue alternating stitching.

Cuffing a Pant Leg

If you can sew a hem, you can add cuffs to pants. It takes $3^1/_2$ inches of fabric beyond the hemline to sew a standard $1^1/_2$-inch pant leg cuff. Start this project by marking the hemline all around with long basting stitches or pins. Then, with pants off, make two markings: the first $1^1/_2$ inches below the hemline (for the hem allowance) and the second, 2 inches below this marking (for the cuff). Hem pants to the top marking. Create cuffs by folding 2 inches of fabric to the outside; then press to create a sharp crease. To keep cuffs from falling, tack at side seams a $^1/_2$ inch below the top of cuff.

Cuff pants only after you're sure they won't shrink any more.

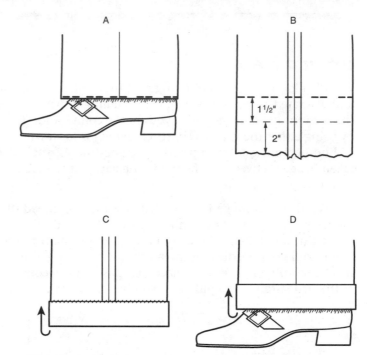

Emergency Measures

What to do when you've got a problem and need a fast fix? Here are quick ways to deal with three of the most common wardrobe uh-ohs:

➤ **Unjamming a zipper**—If it's a plastic coil zipper (not an old-fashioned metal one), fold it crosswise and separate the coil. Close the coil by moving the slider to the bottom stop and then returning it to the top. Rubbing beeswax or candle wax on a stuck zipper helps get it going.

➤ **Stopping a run**—The tried-and-true method is to apply clear nail polish. If you're wearing a pair of dark (black or navy) pantyhose and the run can ruin your chances for, say, getting a job, trying shading your skin underneath the runner with black mascara.

➤ **Reattaching a hem**—If you're in a huge hurry, use a piece of double-stick tape or some safety pins.

Staying Well-Heeled

You may want your footwear to fit as comfortably as an old shoe, but when on the job, you never want to be wearing a pair of shoes that looks anything other than brand-new. Think that's an impossibility? Well, think again. When properly cared for, leather never has to show its age; indeed, even worn leather can be beautifully restored.

Shoe Care: Steps in the Right Direction

Keep your bottom line looking healthy with these tips:

➤ Use nonlacquered wooden shoe trees, which best absorb moisture (that is, perspiration, one of the biggest causes of shoe deterioration), deodorize, and help retain the shape of the shoe.

➤ Add thin, protective, rubber soles to the bottom of leather shoes. Rubber soles improve traction and help keep water from soaking through to the uppers. Since they can extend the life of the soles about three times, you'll want to replace your protective soles as soon as they begin to wear through.

➤ Use a shoehorn when slipping your feet into your shoes. It helps keep the heel *counter* (which is the leather support between the lining and the upper) from losing its stability.

➤ Plastic protectors that are nailed to shoe tips and heels make shoes last longer if those areas are especially prone to wear.

➤ Loosen shoe laces and buckles when removing your shoes to keep them from stretching out of shape.

➤ Treat all new shoes (and handbags, briefcases, and leather jackets) to both a protective coat of paste or cream polish and a non-silicone waterproofing product before wearing or using them. (Stay away from silicone and mink oil, which can significantly darken leather and prevent it from "breathing.") Reapply water repellent as soon as water no longer beads off the leather surface.

➤ Condition smooth leather (handbags, briefcases, jackets, and belts, as well as shoes) every other month with a cream or liquid conditioner to maintain its flexibility and prevent cracking and scratches.

➤ Brush suede often since its nap can flatten and collect dust. Special suede brushes are available, but a toothbrush makes a good stand-in.

➤ Replace soles and heels as they become worn down.

➤ Protect shoes when traveling by packing them in suede bags or old socks.

Do-It-Yourself Restoration

When shoes need some TLC, you don't necessarily have to take them into the shop. There are a number of repairs you can tackle yourself.

Smooth Leather

To restore the luster to a worn pair of leather shoes:

1. Clean the surface with a leather soap, applied with a damp cloth. Wipe the surface with a second cloth moistened with clean water.

2. Apply a wax-based polish with a soft cloth, working it in a circular motion; a colored polish masks scratches and fading, while a neutral polish preserves the surface color.

3. Once polish dries, buff it with a flannel cloth to raise a shine.

To remove an oil or grease stain, blot up as much of the stain as possible and then rub talcum powder into the stain; the powder should absorb most of the stain. Remove the talc with a leather cleaner.

Suede

Suede is leather that's finished by buffing to produce a velvetlike napped surface. Suede is softer, thinner, and therefore not as durable as regular leather.

To renew old suede shoes:

1. Rub out any stains with a suede stone or "eraser" and then brush off dust with a brass-bristle suede brush. (You can get these supplies at shoe-repair stores or wherever shoe-care supplies are sold.)

2. After testing for colorfastness, wash the shoe's surface with a cleanser designed for suede, using a barely damp sponge. Fit shoe trees inside and let the shoes dry overnight.

3. The next day, give the shoes a light brushing to raise the nap.

As an alternative, you can use steam and a suede brush to get rid of scuffs and restore some color. Here's how:

1. Hold your scuffed shoe above a pot of boiling water to raise the nap of the suede.

2. Then, away from the heat, brush the matted suede. If the suede has an oil stain, try talcum powder to absorb it. Leave the powder on overnight and then use your suede brush to lift the nap.

Patent Leather

To remove scuffs from patent leather (leather which is covered with a flexible, water-proof film with a lustrous mirrorlike surface) dampen a soft cloth with vinegar and swab over the shoes. Patent leather also shines up beautifully when it's wiped with Windex.

Leather and the Weather

Though leather is naturally somewhat water-resistant, after a chance encounter with a puddle or a mound of snow, leather shoes require some special treatment. This advice is especially true for suede, which can permanently lose its suppleness if it gets soaked. Make a habit of attending to your wet shoes right away.

➤ Dry your wet shoes at room temperature, never near radiators, fires, or heaters; such intense heat can dry out the leather and cause it to crack.

➤ While your shoes are still damp, insert shoe trees or newspaper to absorb moisture and prevent shoes from curling at the toe.

➤ To remove salt stains, use white vinegar dabbed onto the leather with a clean cloth (follow by wiping with a clean, damp cloth) or wipe with a product made specifically for salt-stain removal. For suedes, gentle cleaning with a suede brush should remove salt residue. If any salt rings still remain, have your shoes professionally cleaned.

Seeking Professional Help

Some jobs (like replacing heels and soles and sewing loose stitching) mandate a visit to the shoe-repair shop. And so do simpler tasks that you know you won't get around to yourself. Considering what you can pay for a pair of shoes or a new briefcase these days, the cost of having a pro maintain your leather accessories is worth it.

Keeping Baubles Beautiful

Whether your jewelry is made of paste or precious metals, you'll want to keep it looking like new. Here's how:

➤ **Gold**—To clean gold jewelry, swish it in a small basin filled with warm soapy water. Use a worn, soft-bristled toothbrush or nailbrush to remove any dirt. Rinse in warm water and dry with a soft cloth. Buffing regularly with a polishing cloth (available for about $5 at jewelry stores) eliminates the need for subsequent washings. To remove scratches, take the item to the store where you bought it. Technicians there should do a free cleaning or polishing with an ultrasonic cleaner.

➤ **Silver**—Clean tarnished silver with silver polish or a polishing cloth specially treated for use on silver. Because of the oils in your skin, frequent wearings help prevent tarnishing and keep silver (and pearls for that matter) glowing.

➤ **Costume jewelry**—Rinse costume jewelry in warm soapy water and use a soft brush where needed. Dry jewelry completely so it won't rust.

A Good Arrangement

How you arrange your closet is your individual decision, based partly on how big it is and how much money you have to spend. (A cadre of companies and professional closet designers will come to your home to help you organize.) A few guidelines, however, should be followed for your clothes' sake:

➤ Don't jam clothes into your closet; ideally, air should circulate around clothing (keeping the closet door ajar helps). If you have a big wardrobe, rotate it seasonally, moving the out-of-season stuff to the back.

The Fashion Police

Line bureau drawers with shelf paper to prevent clothing from coming into contact with the damaging acids in wood, as well as from snagging on splinters. When stacking clothing in drawers or on a shelf, keep lighter items on top of heavier ones to avoid crushing.

➤ Arrange clothing in different categories (pants, jackets, suits, shirts, and so on) to simplify finding things.

➤ Clean clothes before you pack them away for the season. (Previously invisible stains can oxidize over time and become permanent in storage.)

➤ Hang jackets on heavy wooden or molded plastic hangers that fill out the entire width of the shoulders; wire breaks down shoulder pads over time and may leave hard-to-remove creases in thin fabrics. By virtue of their size, more substantial hangers keep clothing spaced farther apart, which minimizes the risk of clothing being crushed.

➤ Button the top few buttons on a garment to keep it hanging straight.

➤ Store knits folded; otherwise, they'll stretch out of shape.

➤ Store out-of-season clothes in your closet in cloth bags to keep them from getting dusty (plastic covers attract dust and prevent natural fabrics from breathing).

➤ Hang suits together on one suit hanger, as both a time- and space-saving device.

➤ Hang pants upside down from the cuffs, folded along the crease line. Remove belts.

➤ Use cedar hangers, blocks, or strips to help keep moths out of closets and drawers and away from the natural fibers on which they love to feast. If you have a separate closet for out-of-season clothes, consider using mothballs or, alternatively, OFF! Moth Proofer, lavender-scented sachets that repel moths for one clothing storage season.

➤ Store at least your good shoes in shoe trees. To protect your shoes from dust, consider keeping them in their original boxes. To make it easier to find the pair you want when you want it, attach a Polaroid picture of the shoes or write a description on the box.

➤ Hang belts from their buckles on a belt hanger or hook.

➤ Store ties on rod racks or revolving tie carousels.

The Least You Need to Know

➤ A well-maintained wardrobe helps enhance your professional image, and vice versa!

➤ Clothing-care labels, which give you instructions about wash–water temperature, whether to line or tumble dry, and when to dry clean, take much of the mystery out of doing laundry. Use them.

➤ A good dry cleaner, like a good tailor, can be found via word of mouth. Ask around.

➤ Being able to perform small clothing-repair tasks, such as mending a fallen hem or sewing on a button, is part of being a good dresser.

➤ The least complicated and most inexpensive alterations are those that only tweak the fit of a garment rather than change it considerably.

➤ Leather shoes and accessories require frequent cleaning, conditioning, polishing, and waterproofing to maintain their suppleness and luster. And the regular use of shoehorns and shoe trees is vital for keeping shoes properly shaped.

➤ For clothing to remain in good shape, it needs to be neatly and carefully stored—either hanging on sturdy hangers or folded on shelves.

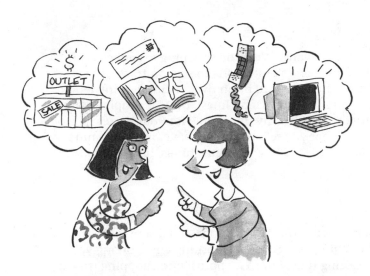

Chapter 23

Talking Shop

In This Chapter

➤ Stores at a glance

➤ Sharpening your shopping skills

➤ A service plan

➤ Beyond department stores

Now that you know what clothing and accessories to wear to work, all that's left is actually going out and buying them. *All*, you say? How could such a tough, time-consuming task be reduced to something so seemingly effortless?

Of course, I jest. I know from firsthand experience that shopping is anything but simple. Though it should be both enjoyable and easy, shopping has evolved into an anxiety-producing activity—and not just for men. Even though women have a leg up when it comes to knowing the shopping ropes (although I suspect that it's more a part of our upbringing than any inherent born-to-shop tendency), many dislike shopping as much as the guys, or at least are turned off by the same negative aspects of it: the crowds, the overwhelming selection, and the exhausting nature of the endeavor, which often leaves you both sore footed and empty-handed.

Since the alternative to shopping, namely, going without appropriate garb, is hardly a viable option, what's needed instead—and provided in this chapter—is a crash course in survival training for shoppers—a rundown of strategies to help you get better service, prevent buying mishaps, and find precisely what you're looking for. And for those looking to stay far away from the maddening crowds of the mall, there's also an overview of outlets that permit shopping in the privacy of your own home.

Shopping Smart

You know the expression the best-laid plans? Well, the shopping experience can certainly throw a monkey wrench into one's best efforts to stay on track. It's no understatement to say that clothes shopping can be an overwhelming experience. Even if you had free run of the stores (no crowds, no lines), there is simply so much merchandise to see, feel, and try on, it's virtually impossible for your senses not to become overloaded. After a while, what you're buying may have little in common with what you actually need. To make it easier to buy the right things, heed the following advice.

Be a Good Scout

Some people—those, like myself, whom I think of as professional shoppers—may relish the idea of arriving at a mall first thing on a Saturday morning and working your way from one end to another until closing time, but that approach to shopping isn't the best one for most amateurs—since the experience can leave you overwhelmed and exhausted.

A better idea, one that makes shopping excursions more productive and less stressful, is to preshop. It's no more complicated than flipping through a couple catalogs, window-shopping on your lunch hour, or casually wandering the aisles of a few stores. All this strategy requires you to do is take some time to look around, familiarize yourself with what's out there (and how much it's selling for) before actually jumping in with both feet.

The beauty of this plan is that it doesn't require a plan: You can scout on a whim and spend as much or as little time at it as you like. It won't cost you a thing—unless you find something perfect, in which case you can buy it or simply make a mental note. Plus, it will remove any pressure to buy; you can simply say to any over-eager sales-people, "No thanks, I'm just looking."

While you're at it, use the time you're scouting in stores to learn the lay of the land. In smaller stores, it's pretty easy to figure out how to get to your destination; most chain stores, like JCPenney and Sears, group all the men's clothes together (sometimes on a separate floor) and all the women's clothes together. Though there's a lot to look at, you don't have to travel that far. Stores like The Gap, Banana Republic, and Eddie Bauer—all great shopping spots for work clothes—seem to have adopted similar floor plans.

It's a totally different story in department stores, in which women's shoes and men's sweaters are often sold in three different departments—often on as many different floors. (Because they're usually situated on just two floors, department stores in malls generally the easiest to navigate.) At the same time, individual designers and brands usually have their own departments—in which more accessories and sweaters are offered. It can be quite confusing especially since no two department stores seem to be laid out the same—which is why these short scouting periods are such a good idea.

The Fashion Police

While you're scouting, don't automatically rule out any stores or departments because you think they're too expensive for your limited budget. Take the opportunity to expand your horizons. Check out mannequins and store displays, to see how the professionals put together outfits. Even if you can't afford to buy anything, you're likely to get inspired by, say, an interesting color combination or style of shoe that you can easily translate into your own look—especially considering the speedy way fashion trends now trickle down from Calvin Klein to Kmart! Plus, you never know what you're going to find on sale.

Don't Be Impulsive

How many items of clothing have you purchased without knowing what you were going to pair them with, or even worse, knowing for a fact that they weren't going to go with anything else you owned? Probably lots. If you're like most people, your closet is filled with lots of misfits—those pieces that aren't part of an outfit or that can't be incorporated into one unless you invest in more clothing. Why are we so prone to buying misfits? Because it's so easy to be seduced by an appealing color, some scrumptuously soft fabric, or a good fit. (We all know what a major victory finding something that fits can be!) Unfortunately, none of these are good enough reasons to buy.

One easy way to minimize the number of misfits you buy is to know in advance what you're shopping for, be it a navy suit or two dress shirts—one white, one blue, possibly with a chalk stripe. Without at least some sort of preconceived notion of what you need, it's easy to fall into the trap of buying on impulse. Another helpful device is the list you created that details what you already own (refer to Chapter 7, "Getting Started"). Carry it with you while shopping and—before you even get close to the cash register—check to see how the garment in question is going to fit in with what you already own.

Love It or Leave It

A friend once summed up her satisfaction with something by saying, "like it, don't love it." When it comes to clothing, you should really love (or at least feel strongly about) whatever it is you're buying—especially when you consider how much money it's costing you. That means it should fit well (or be easily altered) and flatter you to no end. Clothing that plays this role will boost your self-confidence tremendously, while clothing that doesn't can have the opposite effect. And who needs that?

Don't Play the Waiting Game

One of the most common things people do to sabotage their efforts to build a well-coordinated wardrobe is shop at the 11th hour. This is when you're most desperate and, therefore, most willing to overlook everything that matters—quality, cost, fit, and color. Ironically, it's often for the biggest events—a job interview, a speech, the company Christmas party—that you find yourself combing the racks in search of the perfect something to wear. Need it be said that last-minute shopping isn't a good habit to get into?

Good Things Take Time

Just as Rome wasn't built in a day, you shouldn't expect to buy everything you need to complete your wardrobe in a single afternoon. For one thing, you probably can't afford to—either financially or emotionally (when tempted to shop 'til you drop, remember that tomorrow is another day). And anyway, it's better to stock up slowly so that you can get acquainted with just a few new acquisitions at a time.

What does this mean? After making several purchases, take them home and play (yes, play!) with them. Try them on together and then with everything else you already own. Haul out your accessories and work them in. You may be pleasantly surprised at how many hidden outfits you'll discover. On the other hand, you'll find out right away what's needed to complete an outfit.

Service with a Smile

It's one of the biggest headaches of shopping: You're either inundated with sales help or treated as if you have the plague. What you want, of course, is service that falls somewhere in the middle, where no one hovers over you when you're in the mood to browse and yet someone is there to help at the right moment—like when you're in the dressing room and need something in a different size. To ensure getting an appropriate level of service, you need to take control of the situation from the get-go—something you can do by employing these strategies:

➤ Dress well to go shopping. If you look like you have money to spend, sales associates will often swarm.

➤ Once a salesperson approaches you, get his or her name and offer your assurance that you'll ask for him or her when—and if—you need help. Treat salespeople with respect, and you'll be rewarded with excellent service.

➤ If a salesperson doesn't approach you until you've started gathering an armload of clothing, allow him or her to "start a dressing room for you." That action signals other salespeople that you're spoken for—though a truly good salesperson will assist another salesperson's customer, if only so that his or her customer's will receive the same treatment in return. Usually from then on, you'll be well attended to—but not in a pushy way.

➤ If other salespeople continue to approach you, smile politely and say that Mary or John is helping you. Your goal is not to alienate anyone, since Mary or John may be on break by the time you're ready to try things on or have your purchases rung up.

➤ Timing is crucial if you're after good service. Stores are much less crowded Monday through Friday during off-hours (mornings and afternoons) and when sales aren't in full swing. In general, service is better at smaller specialty stores and boutiques.

Your Salesperson, Your Friend?

As a former salesperson in department stores, I know that there are salespeople who want not only to keep up their sale figures, but to genuinely assist customers in finding what they're looking for—and in making purchases they'll be happy with. Then again, I also know that there are sales people who have their own best interest at heart—and the merchandise they sell probably gets returned or exchanged a lot!

A smart consumer has their radar up for the latter, as one of my customers did when I was working in the better dresses department. We were in the fitting room, and I complemented her on how well a coatdress fit, when she look at me suspiciously, and said in the same breath, "Do you think," and "Do you work on commission?" I was thrilled to be able to answer yes to the first question and no to the second.

Though my customer wouldn't have believed it, the advice or comments of a salesperson who works on commission should be discounted or ignored. (Remember that they don't get to keep commission when garments are returned.) So, how can you know whether a salesperson is feeding you a line—or whether you even want his or her advice? Some tips:

> **Dollars & Sense**
>
> Before buying, check a store's return policy. Ideally, you should be able to receive a full refund or a credit to your charge card if you have your receipt and return the item within the allotted time. Weigh carefully whether you want to shop somewhere that offers only store credit. If you shop there frequently, that's one thing; otherwise, a collection of store credit slips can become a big drain on your finances.

➤ Beware those who flatter you too much. Not everything can be *sooooo* you! Better to work with someone who will recommend a different, more flattering, color or style—or she graciously admits defeat, or suggests another department or store, when he or she doesn't have what you need.

➤ Assess how well the salesperson is dressed. If your taste appears to be better than his or hers, say thanks and that you'll think about it.

➤ Suggesting that you need a larger or smaller size or that a garment needs alterations to fit correctly is usually a good sign. Telling you that it's supposed to fit that way isn't.

➤ Directing you to the sales rack when you describe what you're looking for. A good salesperson appreciates every sale, whether the customer is paying full or half price.

Alternative Shop Ops

Being up close and personal with the merchandise in a store certainly has its advantages (you can feel the fabric, check out the workmanship, and try on before buying), but shopping hardly requires a store anymore. Though hitting the racks is still the most popular way to shop, there are a number of don't-have-to-leave-home alternatives that even die-hard store shoppers may want to consider. Here are the top three, along with the information you need to know to shop them smart.

Mail Call

Convenience is the biggest draw of mail-order catalogs. You can peruse and order from them whenever you wish (often times, toll-free 24 hours a day) and then try on merchandise in the privacy of your bedroom—mixing it with pieces you already own and seeing how it works. Although instant gratification isn't possible, the package frequently arrives within three days after you place the order. (Second-day service is usually also available for an extra charge.) Most catalogs charge for shipping and handling—anywhere from about $5 to $15.

The downside to shopping via catalogs is that, no matter how carefully you assess an item to determine whether it's what you're looking for, there's a fair chance it won't fit right, be quite the color you were expecting, or be exactly as pictured or described. In this case, you will have to arrange for a return—which will cost you at least another couple of bucks in postage. If you exchange something for another size, however, shipping is usually free.

Tips for savvy mail shopping:

➤ Pay close attention to the photograph and accompanying description. Examine the model's pose closely: Are his or her arms awkwardly crossed, possibly to hide an unflattering waistband or other poor design feature? Is the garment fully lined (particularly important if that's what you want)? Does it require dry-cleaning? If information that's important to you is left out of the description, ask the operator who assists you; phone representatives often have additional information about fit and care.

➤ If you find a mail-order catalog that really works for you—the clothes fit well and the styling is becoming—stay with it. Just as with clothing lines found in stores, mail-order companies tend to offer a consistent overall style and fit year after year.

➤ Inquire about the return policy. Merchandise purchased by mail is often covered by a generous return policy, one that can be far more relaxed than that of department stores. I personally have returned items that simply didn't work out as planned six months after receiving them—without any hassle.

Catalogs to Check Out

Hundreds of catalogs, including those sent out by department and chain stores, sell clothing. Here are a few that offer a splendid array of career clothes.

Catalog	Customer service
Bachrach (m)	800-637-5840
Banana Republic (w&m)	888-906-2800
Boston Proper (w)	800-243-4300
Brooks Brothers (w&m)	800-274-1815
Chadwick's of Boston (w)	800-525-6650
Clifford & Wills (w)	800-922-1035
Eddie Bauer (w&m)	800-426-8020
AKA Eddie Bauer (w&m)	800-327-8852
Harold's Direct (w&m)	800-676-5373
J. Crew (w&m)	800-444-9449
J. Jill (w)	800-642-9989
The J. Peterman Company (w&m)	800-231-7341
Lands' End (w&m)	800-356-4444
Lands' End Beyond Buttondowns (m)	800-356-4444
Lands' End First Person Singular (w)	800-966-4434
L.L.Bean (w&m)	800-221-4221
Nicole Summers (w)	800-642-6786
Nine West By Mail (w)	800-999-1877
Pendleton Woolen Mills (w&m)	800-760-4844
Spiegel (w&m)	800-345-4500
Talbots (w)	800-825-2687
Tweeds (w)	800-999-7997

m=menswear; w=womenswear

Shopping the Web

No malls. No calls. Such is the beauty of shopping via the Internet. Or at least, in theory, that's the advantage. The reality is that shopping via computer still leaves something to be desired, since not all Web sites permit orders to be placed while you're online. Sometimes you have to call a toll-free number to place an order or mail or fax an order form that you print out from your computer. Also annoying is the limited selection of a manufacturer's or store's offerings for a specific season and the fact that many of the photos aren't of good enough quality to show design details very well (though some sites do have the capability of enlarging the photo with a click of the mouse). There's also a lot of waiting-around time while information gets transferred to your computer—depending on your particular system.

Still, the Internet can be an entertaining way to shop—there's something rather exciting about seeing the site develop before your eyes. That many companies add interesting and informative commentary about everything from building a wardrobe to how to pack for a trip to caring for clothing often makes a visit worthwhile, even if you don't find anything to buy.

Currently, while most Internet users (more than 70 percent) browse product Web sites, only a fraction (15 percent) actually make purchases online, according to a research study. The main reason: concerns about the security of electronic payments.

Tips for savvy online shopping:

➤ Before buying, check with the site's help page to see whether your transactions are being encrypted, or electronically scrambled, for safety.

➤ To steer clear of scams or illegitimate merchants, order only from outfits with an established retail operation. Or if the retailer exists only on the Internet, look for a phone number on the site and call for information about the product and payment choices.

Sites to See

To determine whether Internet shopping is for you, check out some sites. Even if they don't permit you to order online, most give you an idea of the type of merchandise offered by the manufacturer or store, as well as provide telephone numbers to order products and/or request a catalog, store locations, upcoming special events, and even weekly sale items.

Shopping sites	Site features
www.bachrach.com	❏
www.bloomingdales.com	❏ ➤
www.brooksbrothers.com	❏ ➤
www.coat.com (Burlington Coat Factory)	❏ $

Shopping sites	Site features
www.coach.com	X ➤
www.dextershoe.com	X ➤
www.eddiebauer.com	❑ ➤ ➤
www.fashionmall.com	❑
www.gap.com	❑ ➤
www.haroldscatalog.com	❑ ➤ $
www.netpad.com/hushpuppies	❑ ➤
www.jcpenney.com	❑ ➤
www.jcrew.com	❑ $
www.johnstonmurphy.com	❑ X
www.jpeterman.com	❑ ➤
www.kennethcole.com	X ➤
www.kmart.com	X ➤ $
www.landsend.com	❑
www.lanebryant.com	❑ ➤
www.levi.com	❑ ➤
www.lizclaiborne.com	X ➤
www.llbean.com	❑ ➤
www.macys.com	❑ ➤
www.ninewest.com	X ➤
www.pendleton-usa.com	❑ ➤
www.qvc.com	❑
www.rockport.com	X ➤
www.sears.com	X ➤
www.spiegel.com	❑
www.talbots.com	X ➤
www.target.com	X ➤
www.timex.com	❑ ➤
www.todaysman.com	o ➤

❑ = *online shopping; X = browsing only, no shopping;* ➤ *= area store information; $ = sale listings*

Small-Screen Shopping

Home shopping on TV stations such as QVC and the Home Shopping Channel is a huge business; QVC averages 113,000 orders each day, and sales in 1996 reached $1.8 billion!

How does home shopping work? Basically like this: Designers or their spokespeople come on the show for specified periods of time and talk about the clothing being offered that day. They describe in great detail each piece's design features, the fabric, how the item fits, how it's best worn, and whether it's machine washable. Meanwhile, models wearing the clothing appear onscreen. These channels sell accessories in the same way.

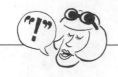

Quote . . . Unquote

Veni, vidi, Visa. (We came, we saw, we went shopping.) ...Jan Barrett

The goal during each segment is to sell every last piece of the merchandise being offered, hence the reason there's sometimes an onscreen tally keeping count of how many of each item still remains in stock. You better hurry, or you'll miss out; it seems to be telling viewers— a ploy that builds excitement and stimulates sales. If you make a mistake when buying, home-shopping networks usually have very reasonable return policies—although, as with mail-order catalogs, the shipping charges can add up.

Tips for savvy TV shopping:

➤ Pay close attention to the information being given by the host, since it can provide necessary clues as to whether the item is correct for you.

➤ Be aware that colors may look different onscreen than they do in real life.

The Least You Need to Know

➤ The quality of your wardrobe is a reflection of your shopping skill. Toward that end, spend some time scouting the stores to learn the terrain, stand firm on quality and fit, shop with a list, and eschew the shopping-spree mentality.

➤ Though it may not always seem as such, a store's sales staff is there to assist you. Even if you don't think you're going to require help (say, perhaps, you really are just browsing), take the name of the first salesperson who approaches you; you never know when you may require some service.

➤ Mail-order catalogs, the Internet, and home-shopping channels are convenient alternatives to shopping in stores, but returns are common because you can't try on the merchandise before you buy.

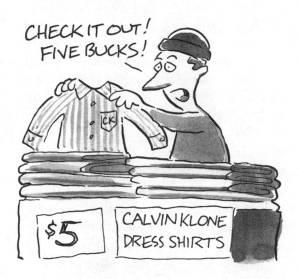

Chapter 24

Investment Dressing on a Budget

In This Chapter

➤ Six steps to a richer-looking wardrobe

➤ Increase your sale savvy

➤ Stores that specialize in savings

➤ Sew it yourself—and save

➤ When to scrimp, when to splurge

It's a common scenario: You want to raise your profile at work by dressing more professionally, but funds are low. How can you upgrade your look when your budget is so limited? That's simple: By hunting down the best bargains, working the sales like a pro, and stretching your dollar to the breaking point. In this chapter, the how-to's on these and other penny-pinching practices.

Cheap, but Chic

No one need know that your outfit didn't cost half your paycheck. By following these pointers, the inexpensive can look downright expensive.

➤ Buy classically styled clothing in dark colors, which can go a long way toward camouflaging inferior design and fabric. Frou-frou detailing, especially in bright or garish colors, rarely looks rich—even if you're paying a lot for it.

Dollars & Sense

Resist the temptation to stuff your closets with oodles of mediocre merchandise. Instead, concentrate on buying a smaller selection of higher-quality, classic-style garments. They may cost more up front, but—since the garments will last for years—be less expensive in the long run.

Fashion Footnote

Most department stores and specialty shops carry their own brand of merchandise (in fashion lingo, it's referred to as *private label*), which often packs a big style punch at a much lower price. Also, if you really like a designer's styling, check out her "secondary" or "bridge" line, which sells for as much as 50 percent less but is styled in the same vein.

➤ Replace run-of-the-mill buttons with ones that are more unusual and/or made of finer materials. Good options are brass, leather, horn, mother-of-pearl, and wood. Add a dash of color by attaching sew-through buttons with thread in a color that contrasts with the garment; such a small, but distinctive touch is rarely seen on off-the-rack clothing.

➤ Opt for less luxurious fabrics, say, rayon or polyester for silk, mimic a more expensive look.

➤ Pair one fabulous garment (ideally, a jacket) with more moderately priced, classically designed, pieces; they'll look more expensive by association.

➤ Tailor your clothes to fit just so and their true pedigree need never be known. Also, be sure clothes are well pressed: After a good ironing, the cheapest rayon shirt, for example, can be as lush and crisp as silk broadcloth.

➤ Substitute a leather belt for the matching one that sometimes comes with a garment. These belts often look so cheap they lower the value of the item—even if it cost a pretty penny.

➤ Remove—and if necessary replace—cardboard or ill-fitting shoulder pads.

Words of Wisdom on Shopping Smart

What's you best advice on shopping on a limited budget? That was the question put to six savvy shoppers—skimpers who dress as though they're big spenders. Here's what they passed on:

➤ "If I can't wear it more than one way, I don't even consider buying it."

➤ "If it's absolutely perfect, I buy it in another color—sometimes, even the same color! It's just so hard to come by something you really like, so when the opportunity presents itself, you've got to take advantage."

➤ "I analyze all my purchases according to a cost-per-wear index. A $300 jacket may sound exorbitant, but if its cost per wear is less than $2 because I'll wear it three times a week, I fork over the bucks."

➤ "I put money into things that get the most use—shoes, jackets, handbags. They'll only go the distance if they're well made."

➤ "I'm not a snob about fabrics. Just because something's made of 60 percent polyester doesn't dissuade me from buying it. If a fabric feels and looks good, that's good enough for me."

➤ "I live by three words: Never pay retail."

Hello, Good Buys

The easiest way to save money when shopping for clothes is obvious: Buy them on sale. In fact, more than a few people interviewed for this book noted that they rarely buy anything for which they pay the suggested retail price—and when they do, it's the perfect something they know they'll wear for years to come.

Still, just because something's on sale is not a good enough reason to buy it. "Bargain clothes" that don't fit correctly, aren't flattering, or don't go with anything else in your wardrobe (and therefore, won't get worn) are anything but bargains—even at half the price.

How do you avoid making such expensive mistakes? Always go shopping with a specific goal in mind (to buy brown pumps, a blue tie, a pair of tan trousers) and don't deviate from the plan—despite the fact that a pink cardigan from Ralph Lauren has been marked down a whopping 75 percent! It's so easy to be blinded by dollar signs and designer labels. Always ask yourself, if a garment was full price and the label had fallen out, would you still want it?

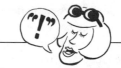

Quote . . . Unquote

Shop early; supplies are limited. ...Store flyer

Dollars & Sense

Stores that have their own charge cards often offer 10 percent off of items bought the day you sign up for one. That's a good deal, but only if you pay off the balance in full when it comes due—since the interest charges are frequently close to 20 percent.

Sales: A Month-by-Month Guide

The easiest way to catch a great sale is to know when stores are most likely to be having one—or at least beginning one, since reductions on many items start one month and continue through the next, until they reach rock-bottom clearance prices. Here are the prime times to shop for whatever you're in the market for.

> **January**—winter coats, high-quality sweaters, winter accessories (gloves, scarves, hats), furs

Fashion Footnote

Technically, a *sale* is a temporary markdown; the price should go back up after the sale ends. A *clearance* is permanent; the price has nowhere to go but down. Unsold sale items often become clearance items.

February—fine jewelry, winter shoes and boots

March—spring preseason sales on suits and separates, spring coats and raincoats, handbags

April—silks and other dressy separates, spring dresses, spring raincoats

May—spring shoes

June/July—swimwear, casual shorts and T-shirts, summer dresses

August—fall pre-season sales on suits and separates

September—back-to-school sales, lined raincoats, better blazers, leather accessories (handbags, wallets)

October—fall suits, career and casual sweaters, winter coats, raincoats and leather jackets

November—fall shoes and boots, eveningwear

December—fine jewelry, cashmere sweaters

On the Hunt: Frequenting New Haunts

There are so many places to shop for bargains if you know where to look for them. Here is a rundown of less traditional retail outlets that can help you save a few bucks— or more.

What's Old Is New Again

Consignment stores and thrift shops both sell used clothing. Between the two, however, you're more likely to find better-quality—albeit pricier—goods at consignment stores, the outlets for clothes and accessories that no longer fit or are no longer wanted but that are still in good condition. Unlike at thrift shops (like the Salvation Army and Goodwill), where clothing ranging from the never worn to the barely wearable is donated and sold at very low prices (with the proceeds usually going to charity), at consignment stores, the owner of the store and seller of the clothes split the profits— thus ensuring that clothing is consistently in shipshape.

The secret to the success of shopping at both consignment or thrift stores is being willing to paw through racks and racks, and tables and tables, of merchandise that's often not well displayed or organized. But sometimes it can be worth it; stories abound of shoppers discovering designer suits at a fraction of their original cost, as well as other famous-name finds. (On a recent trip to Savers, a growing chain of thrift department stores, I found an extremely stylish, like-new Liz Claiborne handbag for $30, while my sister has found a pair of LizSport pants for $9.99.)

The key to second-hand shopping is going in with the right attitude: You just might snap up something wonderful that you otherwise couldn't afford, or—in the case of, say, an antique pin or watch—couldn't even find in a regular store. To get the best merchandise, it pays to be consistent; it's the inveterate shopper, the one who frequently checks the new stock, who often walks away with the best bargains.

Before buying any clothes, be sure to try them on (return policies aren't very buyer-friendly at these stores) and inspect every garment for stains, holes, and other signs of wear—keeping in mind what's fixable and what's not and then factoring in the cost of the repair. Don't be afraid to dicker with the store manager either. One women recently negotiated a handbag marked $40 down to $25 because it was slightly damaged—and then had it fixed for $8!

Off Price Means Low Prices

As T.J. Maxx, an off-price store with a national presence, used to advertise, you get the max for the minimum at its stores. And so it is with all off-price stores. Generally packed with low to moderately priced clothing and accessories, sold at an average of 30 percent less than retail, off-price stores (Filene's Basement, Daffy's, and Marshalls are two other chains) are well organized and usually stocked with plenty of in-season merchandise.

Discounts at the Discount Store

If you only think of stores like Kmart, Caldor, and Target when you need lawn chairs and shampoo, think again. Not only are these discounters an ideal stop for stocking up on the essentials (underwear and pantyhose), they're more than worth a look for basics, especially those with a sportier bent, and for trendy items you may wear for only a short time.

Dollars & Sense

It's not unusual to find clothing, especially hosiery, marked "irregular" at a discount store. Don't let this label discourage you, however. All too frequently, the defect or irregularity isn't noticeable—or is barely so. Just look closely before buying.

The Fashion Police

Think twice about trying to fool people with your designer imposters—those handbags, belts, and scarves, often hawked on street corners or at hole-in-the-wall shops. Unless the fake looks pretty convincing (some do, others don't), it's you who could end up looking foolish. Caveat emptor!

The Outlets: Are They Worth the Trip?

It used to be that there were just a handful of outlet stores (including Loehmann's); now, practically every major brand and designer has its own—which is often represented in one of the more than 400 outlet malls across the country. The question is: Can you save money by shopping at these stores—which are usually located a good distance (at least 25 miles away) from regular malls or urban areas?

In a word, sometimes.

Whereas some outlet stores are the final resting place for irregulars, seconds, overruns, or leftover clothing that mainstream stores couldn't sell, a frequently high percentage of the merchandise is manufactured specifically to stock the outlets—with quality and styling that's sometimes not on par with the brand's (or the designer's) regular line. Since the consumer usually doesn't know whether this merchandise was ever intended to be sold in regular stores (despite the price comparison often heralded on the tag), he or she has to be able to judge a garment on its own merits—not for its label. Unless you've seen a specific garment in, say, a department store, at a much higher price, don't assume you're necessarily getting a deal. Often, if you wait long enough, the sales at regular stores are better than the "reduced" price at outlet stores.

Sample a Sample Sale

Sample sales and stock sales are held at the end of a season to sell overstocks of clothing, as well as those created for promotional purposes. (Clothing photographed in catalogs and magazine are referred to as samples.) Sales are held not long after collections are sold to stores, so the clothes are still in season. Though the selection can be spotty or spectacular (you never know until you arrive), and not all merchandise is available in all colors and sizes, the savings—clothing is sold at wholesale, or about 50 percent the cost of retail—is tremendous.

These sales are usually only held in cities—Atlanta, Chicago, Dallas, Los Angeles, Seattle, and New York—with an apparel mart or manufacturer showrooms. Call the mart and manufacturers in the cities nearest to you to inquire about sale dates.

A Stitch in Time Saves

If you know how to sew, you can easily shave off half, and sometimes more, of the retail price of a garment—even if you choose luxurious fabrics and designer patterns. Provided you have a sewing machine (or access to one), the savings are guaranteed to be substantial. To wit: The sum total required to make a man's 100 percent wool sport jacket (including the pattern, thread, buttons, and other notions), would be about between $75 and $100. In the store, a similar quality jacket would cost, on sale, about $179. That's a difference of at least $75.

Doing it yourself also ensures that a garment will fit you well (altering a pattern isn't that difficult to begin with, and today's patterns are designed to make it even easier) and will be just what you had in mind. How many times have you found the "perfect" outfit in a store—if only it was blue instead of purple, had a different collar, was a tad longer, and came in wool? With home sewing, because you're also acting as the designer, the finished product will fit your exact specifications.

Think your talents with a needle and thread aren't up to snuff? Usually a garment looks homemade only if you go beyond the limitations of your skill. Stick to easy styles (slim skirts, pants, and sheaths are simple to sew), and your efforts will usually be rewarded. Pattern companies have also embraced the novice sewer, producing patterns for all levels of proficiency. Many for beginners combine chic styling and easy construction techniques.

Fashion Footnote

Sewing classes are usually available at high schools for a very low fee. If a needle and thread just isn't for you, maybe a seamstress is. Good seam-stresses often offer their services at very reasonable prices and turn out beautifully finished products—provided you're good at giving direction.

If your biggest reason for not sewing is that you don't have the time, think about how many hours you spend shopping. Whether it's cruising the mall or flipping through catalogs, shopping can easily eat up an evening. Sometimes, particularly when you know what you're after, sewing can actually save you time.

Sound Investments

Expensive isn't always better or necessary. Unless a portion of what you're spending goes to upgrading the fit, feel, and look of a garment, it may not be worth spending the money. Below, the wardrobe assets deserving—and not—of a big capital outlay.

Skimp On...	Splurge On...
Cotton T-shirts	Wool sweater
Hosiery/socks	Leather shoes
Khakis and jeans	Wool trousers
A plain white shirt	A silk camp-style shirt
Trendy jewelry	Fine jewelry or good fakes in classic styles

The Least You Need to Know

➤ Inexpensive clothing looks far pricier when it's classically styled and fits perfectly.

➤ A sale item is only a bargain when it's something you really need.

➤ Sweet deals can often be found at second-hand and consignment stores, where like-new clothing and accessories are sold for a fraction of their original price.

➤ The merchandise available at outlet stores is often manufactured specifically for those stores, and frequently doesn't offer a real savings.

➤ Sewing a garment yourself often saves you at least 50 percent off the retail price of a comparable item.

➤ All clothing and accessories aren't worth a splurge. Skimp on anything trendy or so basic that no one will otherwise know the difference.

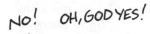

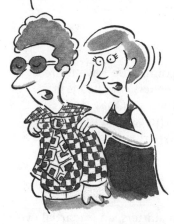

Chapter 25

Need More Help?

In This Chapter

➤ Consulting with the image makers

➤ One-on-one shopping assistance

➤ On the runway

➤ Check the periodicals

➤ Friends, mentors, co-workers

If you've come this far in the book, you must have been inspired by its look-good-to-get-ahead message. And hopefully, you've already started implementing the advice it contains. However, I can imagine lots of scenarios in which you may be ready to jump in with both feet but still be in need of some sort of outside support.

For instance, you may be returning to work after a decade-long hiatus and just don't know where to begin. Or you're just starting out on a very limited budget and can't afford to make any mistakes. Or no matter how familiar you are with the principles of putting together a successful look, you're simply not confident enough in your ability to act on the knowledge. "I know lots of people who have a real knack for dressing and always make a great presentation. Unfortunately, I'm not one of them," says one woman, who jokingly chalks it up to faulty genetic material.

If any of these descriptions are hitting home, don't worry; this chapter discusses a number of strategies for getting more help—including working with professionals whose sole purpose is to help clients implement the very concepts you've been reading about. In addition, there are easy-to-access sources that will further inspire and instruct you in the area of professional dress.

Want a New Image?

Andre Aggasi may say that image is everything, but for those of us who have more conventional careers, it's probably more precise to say that a *professional* image is everything. If you're concerned that your image is less than that, you may want to consider using the services of an image consultant, a person who can advise you on how to update, refine, or make over your look so that it's in synch with the one you're striving for.

What Are Image Consultants?

Just what do you get when you hire an image consultant? For starters, an impartial eye and a good ear, which allow them to honestly assess your sartorial situation and listen carefully to your concerns and objectives. Maybe, for instance, you don't think you're being taken seriously enough at work and want to project more authority.

Though consultants may include different services in their packages, many offer some form of color analysis (the selection of clothing and accessory hues flattering to your hair and skin tones; see Chapter 10, "So Many Options!"); an evaluation of your body by shape, size, and proportion; an overview of what clothing, accessories, hairstyle, and makeup will prove most flattering and effective; and even a closet analysis and cleaning—a professional version of what you read about in Chapter 7, "Getting Started." Some consultants will shop with or for you, while others only advise you on what to buy. Don't worry if you're on a limited budget; many clients are. And what such clients often most appreciate is the advice they get about how to maximize their existing wardrobe with a few new pieces while staying within a small budget.

Dollars & Sense

Can't afford an image consultant? Consider a group consultation. Though you may sacrifice individual attention, you will still get good basic information on style, fit, and color. Plus, the group environment may be less intimidating than a private session. If co-workers are interested, stress the presentation payoff to your boss, and urge him or her to have the company pick up the tab.

Contacting a Consultant

To find a good consultant, ask around; as with everything else, word of mouth is the best referral. You can also check the Yellow Pages under "Image Consultants" or call the Association of Image Consultants International, a professional organization with more than 600 members, at 800-383-8831, to receive a list of local members. A consultant's membership in this organization is considered a must, since there are no licensing or certification requirements in this profession.

Once you've made contact with a consultant, interview her—and I do mean her; most professionals in this area are women, and about 30 percent handle both male and female clients. Some key questions to ask:

➤ How long have you been in business?

➤ What are your fees? (Anywhere from $50 to $175 an hour is standard, with initial consultations ranging from no charge to a steep $250.)

➤ Where did you receive your training? (Ideally, you're looking for training in a course that took more than just a week to complete!)

➤ What's included in the process? (All or just some of what's discussed above?)

➤ Do you specialize? (Some consultants do, in areas like plus sizes, corporate looks, or over-40 clients.)

> **Fashion Footnote**
>
> If your company sends you to see an image consultant, don't be offended—everyone from senators to television newscasters have received some advice. (Some companies actually pay for each new employee to have a consultation!) Instead, consider it an opportunity to hone your skills at making a professional presentation and take the company's willingness to make such a financial investment as a sign of its commitment to you.

➤ Can I speak to two of your clients? (Since you need to feel comfortable with your consultant, ask other clients about her personality and approach.)

Shopping with a Pro

Personal shoppers are a real boon for busy or baffled men and women. What is a personal shopper? "We're a shopping service. We shop the stores for our clients," says one of these pros, who will scout the entire store to find garments that meet your needs and have them ready when you arrive. In reality, however, personal shopping, a little-taken-advantage-of service provided to men and women free of charge by a host of department and specialty stores, goes beyond simply shopping.

Besides all the time saving and amenities (which usually include posh private dressing rooms and complimentary beverages), working with a private shopper generally ensures that you'll receive some frank opinions—though they may be delivered with a soft touch. "She's very candid with me, telling me what does or doesn't work, and I really appreciate her honesty," notes one executive about her personal shopper. That a personal shopper may also clue you in to a style that works great on you but that you never would have picked out yourself can make both your days.

The Personal Shopping Experience

If you're waiting to hear what the catch is to using a personal shopper, you'll be happy to know that there really isn't one. Working with a personal shopper is as easy as

311

filling out a questionnaire so that she (and like image consultants, most personal shoppers are women) can get to know your likes and dislikes. Then you simply call to set up an appointment, give her a general idea of what you'd like to see, and she'll have it in the fitting room ready for you to try on. If the size isn't right, she'll find you another—even if that means calling every store branch.

Personal shoppers aren't exclusive to certain departments, such as the pricey designer boutiques. They'll pick from the sales rack, if that's what it takes. "What sets us apart from other salespeople is that we're knowledgeable about the entire store. That's how we know where some little treasure is going to be," reports one personal shopper.

That knowledge is what makes them so valuable. "I've tried shopping on my own, but I get overwhelmed," notes one executive. "What I like about working with a personal shopper is that I come out with a head-to-toe outfit that works in a lot of different ways." In fact, this woman's new outfit even works with her existing wardrobe, since shoppers keep track of what their clients have already bought. To give them the whole picture, you can even bring in your other clothes—and some reportedly have brought in most of their closets!

Fashion Footnote

The term *personal shopper* may have been coined by Jacqueline Kennedy in a letter she wrote to a hat saleswoman at New York City's Bergdorf Goodman department store. "Could I use you as my personal shopper there?" asked the soon-to-be First Lady.

Unlike image consultants, who shouldn't have any affiliation with a store or clothing company, personal shoppers are still salespeople. But they seem to be bound by the creed, Exert no pressure. The two biggest misconceptions that people have about personal shoppers are that you have to spend a lot of money and that you always have to buy. Not so. They work with all budgets—$50 to $500 and up—and expect that sometimes things just won't work out.

Probably the only downside to working with a personal shopper is that it can take a few visits to get on the same wavelength. But, by all reports, the payoff usually more than makes up for any slow start.

Where the Shoppers Are

Though not always available in all branches, the following stores offer personal shopping services: Macy's, Nordstrom, Bloomingdale's, Saks Fifth Avenue, Bergdorf Goodman, Barneys, and Neiman Marcus. Call your local department store to see whether it offers this service.

Show Me

Fashion shows put on by stores and malls are entertaining ways to see the season's newest clothes and accessories and get inspired by the creative ways they're presented. One thing I really love about these special events, which sometimes feature menswear, is that the clothing being shown is always available at the participating store(s)—which means that you don't have to look any further to buy something you loved.

Sometimes these shows revolve around a specific topic, such as dressing for casual workdays or camouflaging figure problems. And they're emceed by a wardrobe consultant or other fashion expert who usually offers general tips and advice that will apply to your own existing wardrobe, not just the clothes on the runway. To find out about fashion shows in your area, check the newspaper or mall flyers for notices. But be aware that these events may be advertised only to special customers, such as those who have a store charge account.

Fashion Footnote

What's driving more and more men to personal shoppers is the dressing down of business. "Men get the dressy side of business okay, but not the casual. They often think it means jeans and a T-shirt, not a gabardine trouser, button-down shirt, and sweater," notes one personal shopper.

Read All About It

Magazines and newspapers frequently dispense savvy advice about professional dressing, often in columns devoted to job-related issues. Even more helpful is when publications show appropriate clothing and then provide purchasing information. (FYI: If this clothing often seems somewhat pricey, it's because the companies that are best geared to working with fashion editors are frequently those that manufacture moderately and higher-priced clothing. Alternatively, editors may need to feature the clothing of the magazine's advertisers or may simply want to showcase a hot line—regardless of whether the reader can afford or easily find it.)

My gripe with a handful of these widely circulated publications has to do with how frequently the editors undermine the serious tone of such a story by following it up with a wholly ridiculous fashion portfolio that's photographed in an office setting and titled something like, "What You'll Be Wearing to Work This Fall." In more cases than not, the outrageous (or outrageously styled) clothing shown in these stories is hardly representative of any office attire most of us have ever seen—and hopefully, never will.

Free for the Asking

I have a friend whose husband works in a predominantly male office, where a lot of emphasis is put on how employees dress. As she explains it, "These guys are very up front with each other. They have no problem telling someone that his tie is too loud, his shirt isn't pressed enough, or his suit is ugly!" Though it might be hard on the ego, there's certainly an advantage to finding out that your presentation is or isn't working—and learning how to improve it. If you don't have an entire office of Mr. Blackwells to advise you, here are some other sources to consider turning to:

➤ **A co-worker**—When a source of good advice on successful dressing is as close as the next cubicle, try to take advantage of it. There are two ways to gain insight from a well-turned-out co-worker. The first, to observe and emulate his or her style of dress is the best course of action if you're not on comfortable, friendly terms with each other. The second is to simply tell your co-worker how great he/she always looks (a sincere compliment is extremely flattering), to ask where he/she shops, and to ask whether you could go along on a shopping trip. A modified version of this option for those (read men) who aren't comfortable with the straightforward approach, is to inquire less directly about a co-worker's clothing. "Great jacket, where'd you get it?" is a fine opening line.

➤ **A friend**—A real friend won't just gush when you look great; he or she will bite the bullet and tell you—at least when directly asked—when something about your appearance may be holding you back. Maybe a new hairstyle is in order, or perhaps your wardrobe has taken a wrong turn somewhere along the line. Remember your partner in crime from Chapter 7? Ask him or her for an honest appraisal or opinion.

➤ **Your mentor**—Lucky you if you have an older friend or associate who offers you sage career advice. One of the best things about having a mentor is that he or she can be a sounding board, someone you can bounce ideas, concerns, or general questions off of—even if they're about something as seemingly mundane as your wardrobe or hairstyle. Remember: These are people who've been there, done that; and they'll recognize just how important these issues can be.

The Least You Need to Know

➤ Image consultants will, for a fee, help refine or revamp your look.

➤ Personal shoppers are a service provided free to all customers, no matter how much—or how little—money they have to spend.

➤ Friends, co-workers, colleagues, and mentors can be good sources of advice on how to dress successfully.

Glossary

Accent Colors   Vivid or contrasting colors used to break up the monotony of neutrals and provide a bit of zip.

Acetate   A man-made fiber with natural roots. Used during World War I to make waterproof varnishes, today it's called into action when a lightweight, silky fabric is needed. Fabrics made of 100 percent acetate are often used to line garments.

Acrylic   A strong, warm fabric that drapes well, acrylic is often used as a synthetic substitute for wool.

Alpaca   Fleece derived from the alpaca, a member of the camel family that's bred in Peru. Fabrics made from alpaca are warm and lightweight, with a silky, soft hand and good draping properties.

American-Cut Suit   A conservative-style suit, often called the sack suit. It's single-breasted, boxy, and fashioned with little shoulder padding and a single, centered back vent.

Apron   The wide end of a tie.

Argyle   A multicolored, diamond pattern knitted into socks and sweaters.

Ballistic Nylon   Nylon fabric that's so strong, perforations don't tear it. Frequently used in luggage.

Balmacaan   A loose-fitting coat noted for its raglan sleeves, small collar, and button front. Frequently made of nubby tweed and smooth, worsted wool. It's named for an estate near Inverness, Scotland.

Banded Collar   A dress shirt with a band of fabric in place of a collar.

Barrel Cuffs   Shirt cuffs that close with a button.

Bemberg Lining   A type of lining fashioning from a silky soft type of rayon. It's most frequently used in fine menswear.

Besom Pocket   An interior pocket bound by strips of fabric, called welts.

Blazer   In its purest and most versatile form, a solid, dark jacket made of medium-weight fabric. The original blazer, which was navy blue with brass buttons, was part of the British naval uniform.

Blended Yarns   Those that combine the most desirable features of several fibers. For instance, one very common match-up, a wool/polyester blend, combines the drapability of wool and the strength and wearability of polyester.

Body   The term used to describe the solid, compact feel of fabrics.

Box Pleats   Double pleat formed by two facing folds.

Break   A term that refers to the slight fold created in the neat line of the crease in pants when the fabric skims the top of the shoe.

British-Cut Suit   A style of suit that adheres to the lines of the body. It has softly padded shoulders, a nipped-in waist, and side vents.

Broadcloth   Both a closely woven wool-suiting cloth with a smooth nap and lustrous appearance, and a tightly woven cotton or cotton-blend cloth with a fine crosswise rib that's frequently used for shirts.

Button-down Collar   That which is secured to the shirt by two small buttons at the collar points.

Cable Knit   A raised, decorative pattern resembling twisted cables that's frequently used in sweaters.

Camel Hair   The thick, soft undercoat of the Bactrian camel of Asia.

Camp Shirt   A style of shirt distinguished by two patch or flap pockets and a convertible collar.

Cardigan   A button-down sweater named after the seventh earl of Cardigan, who wore such a sweater under his military uniform.

Cashmere   The fine, downy-soft undergrowth that grows on the cashmere goat.

Chalk Stripe   White stripes of varying widths that resemble chalk lines.

Challis   A lightweight, plain woven fabric printed with a delicate floral pattern; mostly used as a dress fabric.

Chambray   Sort of a lightweight denim, it's woven with colored and white threads. A popular shirting fabric, chambray was originally woven in Cambrai, France.

Check   The term for all patterns made of crossing stripes.

Chesterfield   A semifitted, straight-cut coat in a single- or double-breasted style, usually with a black velvet collar. Introduced in the 1940s as a man's coat by the fourth earl of Chesterfield, it fits much like an elongated blazer.

Clarity   A term that refers to a color's brightness.

Clearance   A sale to clear out stock. The reduced price will never be raised.

Coatdress   A dress styled like a coat.

Consignment Store   One that sells used clothing. At consignment stores, the owner of the clothing and the owner of the store share the profits.

Convertible Collar   A collar that can be worn open or fastened by a small, concealed button and loop. When closed, a convertible collar resembles a spread or straight collar.

Cool Colors   Those with blue undertones.

Corduroy   From the French *corde du roi*, or "cloth of the king," a durable fabric characterized by wide wales, pinwales, cords, or ribs.

Cotton   A natural fiber that comes from the seed hairs of the cotton plant.

Cotton, carded   A process that removes most of the impurities and a certain amount of short or broken fibers.

Cotton, combed   Cotton that has undergone an extra step beyond carding, in which all the short fibers are removed. Combing produces yarn that's softer and more lustrous, even, and compact than carded cotton.

Cotton, Pima   A fine, long-staple cotton.

Cotton, Sea Island   The finest grade of cotton.

Crease or Wrinkle Resistance   A finish used on cotton, linen, rayon, and blended fabrics that increases resistance to and recovery from wrinkling.

Crepe   Any fabric with a crinkly, pebbly surface. (The word crepe comes from the French term *crépu*, meaning crimped or crinkled.) Crepe has a dressy feel, drapes well, and is good at resisting wrinkles.

Crewneck   A round neckline often finished with knit ribbing.

Cuffs   The folded end of a pant leg.

Dart   A construction device used to build a definite shape into a flat piece of fabric so that the fabric conforms to a particular body contour or curve.

Denier   A numbering system in which low numbers represent fine yarn sizes and high numbers indicate coarser, heavier sizes—and consequently, stronger, more durable fabric.

Denim   A rugged, cotton twill fabric, denim comes in many colors other than the original indigo blue. Its name is derived from Nîmes, France, the town in which it originated.

Drape   Describes the way a fabric falls when hung or arranged in different positions.

Dry Cleaning   A waterless process in which a liquid solvent and a detergent pass continually through the clothes, dissolving dirt and stains. Unlike water, the solvent won't cause dyes to bleed or run, is unlikely to cause shrinkage, and won't wash out details like pleats.

317

Duffel   A short or long woolen coat with a hood that hangs straight from the shoulders and fastens with toggles, rather than buttons. It was worn by men in the British navy during World War II and adapted as a sport coat for men and women in the 1950s. You'll find it in wool and wool blends and in sporty plaid fabrics. It's named for the fabric, a heavy napped woolen originally made in Duffel, Belgium. This style, which is also called a stadium coat, is ideal when paired with casual work clothes.

Fabric   Cloth made by the interlacing of yarns of fiber.

Fashion or Costume Jewelry   That which is made of plated metals, as well as other materials, such as cubic zirconia, glass, plastic, and rhinestones.

Fiber   The basic component of fabric. Fibers can be derived from natural sources such as plants or animals, or synthesized from chemicals.

Fine Jewelry   That which is made from precious metals like gold, sterling silver, and platinum, often in combination with precious or semiprecious stones.

Flannel   A softly brushed fabric, often made of worsted wool, that lends a casual, sporty look to blazers or trousers.

Flap Pocket   An interior pocket with a flap that covers its opening. When placed on an angle, a flap pocket is called a hacking pocket.

Flat Front   A skirt or pant without pleats.

Floral   Any pattern in which flowers predominate.

Fly Front   When buttons are hidden by a placket; very common on jeans and coats.

Foulard   A small geometrical design on a plain background.

Four-in-Hand Knot   A small, straight knot that can be adjusted to fit any collar style. It is the most commonly used knot for tie tying.

French Cuffs   A double cuff that folds back over itself and is usually fastened with a cuff link.

Full Fashioned   A technique of knitting in which fabric panels are shaped during the knitting process by increasing or decreasing the number of loops. Full-fashioned garments will fit better, have less-prominent seams, and—as a result—be more expensive than those that are "cut and sewn," a technique in which panels are cut from a bolt of knit cloth and then sewn together.

Fusing   Interfacing that is glued to the outer fabric.

Gabardine   A durable, tightly woven fabric with definite diagonal ridges that can be made in a variety of weights from natural and synthetic fibers. It's the workhorse of suiting fabrics and can be made of wool, cotton, or a blend of fibers.

Gathering   A method in which a large amount of material is drawn into a smaller space, creating soft, even folds—usually at a waistband or shirt cuff.

Gauntlet Button   The button situated several inches above the cuff of the sleeve, designed to keep the sleeve opening closed.

Gingham   A usually cotton fabric with stripes of equal width in two colors, one of which is generally white. The stripes intersect to create squares and a third color that's a blend of the other two.

Glen Plaid   A pattern characterized by two checks of different sizes. It was named for Glen Urquhart, a valley in Invernesshire, Scotland.

Hacking Pocket   *See flap pocket.*

Half-Windsor Knot   A downsized Windsor knot, used to tie a tie.

Hand   A reference to the way a fabric feels, that is, soft or stiff.

Herringbone   A pattern with a sideways zigzag or chevron effect.

Houndstooth   A pattern of even, broken checks, frequently in black and white.

Image Consultant   A professional who can advise you on how to update, refine, or make over your look.

Inseam   The length in inches of the inside of the leg, from the crotch to the leg bottom.

Inside Lines   Those based on a garment's construction and ornamentation. Lapels, collars, pleats, tucks, zippers, pockets, belts, plackets, and seams are examples of inside lines.

Interlock Knit   A fine-gauge fabric in which the front and back of fabric looks identical.

Italian-Cut Suit   A style of suit that fits snugly and has high, padded shoulders. The jackets are generally unvented.

Jersey   A soft, smooth, stretchable fabric without a distinct rib.

Kelly Bag   A handbag originally designed by the French fashion house Hermès and named for Grace Kelly.

Keyhole Buttonhole   A buttonhole shaped like a keyhole. The enlarged resting place for the button ensures that the buttonhole will not be distorted when the garment is buttoned.

Khaki   A sturdy material, historically used for military uniforms, that's a dull yellowish-brown color.

Khakis   A style of pant that rules on casual Fridays; also referred to as chinos.

Lambswool   Wool that comes from the first shearing of a lamb; it's very soft and has wavy fibers.

Lapel   The turned-back front section of a jacket, coat, or shirt, where this section joins the collar. Notched and peaked are two common lapel shapes.

Linen   Fibers and fabric derived from the flax plant.

Lining   Most often made from a relatively slippery fabric, a lining is applied to the inside of a garment to hide its inner construction. Linings add warmth to a garment and make it easier to put on and take off.

Loafer   A slip-on shoe with a covered instep.

Mercerization   Process in which cotton is treated with caustic soda to give a silky, lustrous finish that helps to increase its strength.

Merino Wool   A fine, high-quality wool yarn derived from Merino sheep.

Microfiber   Polyester or nylon fibers that, as their name implies, have much smaller diameters than their traditional counterparts.

Mohair   A long, white, lustrous hair obtained from the Angora goat. (The fabric referred to as angora actually comes from the Angora rabbit.)

Moleskin   A heavy, strong cotton fabric brushed to suedelike softness.

Monkstrap   A slip-on shoe with a buckled strap across the instep.

Monochromatic   One color, head to toe. Dressing monochromatically makes you appear taller and slimmer.

Neutrals   Colors like black, gray, navy, and beige that are more versatile and less memorable than brights or pastels.

Nylon   A high-strength, quick-drying, elastic fiber.

Off-Price Stores   Those that sell low- to moderately priced clothing and accessories at an average discount of 30 percent less than retail.

Outlet Store   Traditionally, the final resting place for irregulars, seconds, overruns, or leftover clothing that manufacturers couldn't sell to mainstream stores. Today, a frequently huge percentage of merchandise is manufactured specifically to stock these stores—albeit with quality and styling that's sometimes not on par with a brand's (or the designer's) regular line.

Outseam   The length in inches of the outside of the leg, from the waist to the bottom of the pant leg.

Oxford   Any shoe that ties. Cap-toe oxfords have an extra layer of plain or perforated leather across the toes; plain-toe oxfords have no extra decoration.

Oxford Cloth   A durable fabric woven from heavy, predominantly cotton, yarns. Button-down shirts are frequently made of oxford cloth.

Paisley   A curvy pattern of amoeba-like shapes that was derived from the shape of the date palm tree.

Patch Pocket   A pocket sewn onto the outside of a garment.

Patent Leather   Leather covered with a flexible, waterproof film with a lustrous mirrorlike surface.

Pattern   A design that's woven into, or printed onto, fabric.

Pencil Stripe   A dark, narrow stripe on a lighter background.

Personal Shopper   A store employee who assists customers with their shopping needs. Personal shopping is a free service.

Pills   Surface fibers that have rolled up into tiny balls due to friction.

Pinstripes   Very narrow lines (the width of a straight pin) created by a succession of dots.

Piqué   A durable, knitted cotton fabric with a waffle or diamond-shaped pattern that's produced by weaving together two cloths, one above the other. Polo shirts are often fashioned of piqué.

Plaid   A pattern is technically a plaid, which means blanket in Gaelic, when colored stripes or bars cross each other at right angles and form squares or blocks.

Plain Weave   The simplest and most commonly used weave, accounting for 80 percent of woven fabrics. Its effect resembles a checkerboard pattern.

Pleats   Folds in the fabric that release to accommodate fullness.

Ply   The term refers to the number of strands twisted to form a single yarn. The higher the number (usually one to four), the plusher, warmer, and thicker the garment.

Pocket Square   A piece of fabric used to adorn a handkerchief pocket.

Polka Dots   Round spots of any size; the most common version is white dots on a colored background.

Polo Coat   Double- or single-breasted, the polo coat often comes in camel hair or camel-colored wool. It has a long, slightly fitted cut, patch pockets, and, usually, a half belt in back.

Polo Shirt   A pullover with a rolled collar and anywhere from one to four buttons at the neck, it was originally worn to play polo.

Polyester   One of the most frequently used synthetic fibers in clothing; it keeps its shape, resists creasing, wears well, and is a breeze to care for.

Poplin   A strong, hard-wearing fabric used mostly for high-quality shirting and summer suits, it's characterized by crosswise ribs that give it a corded effect.

Preshrinking   A process to inhibit further shrinkage.

Pullman   The rectangular case (basically a box with a hinged lid) that has long been synonymous with the word *suitcase*. Pullmans with special compartments designed to hold your suits or dresses are known as "suiters."

Pump   A slip-on shoe that reveals the foot's instep.

Rayon   A synthetic fiber or fabric composed of a material derived from trees and plants. Rayon was originally dubbed "artificial silk."

Reefer   A takeoff of the British naval coat, it's a double-breasted, semifitted coat with notched lapels and a double row of buttons in the front.

Regimental Stripes   Diagonal stripes, so called because they were worn by English regiments in certain identifying colors.

Reprocessed Wool   Wool that's been previously woven, but not worn.

Reweaving   A process in which a missing area of a garment is painstakingly recreated so that the weave and pattern are duplicated exactly via tiny, precise stitches.

Rib Knit   Fabric with lengthwise ribs of any width; rib knitting is heavier and more durable and elastic (especially in the crosswise direction) than flat knitting—making it especially suitable for cuffs and waistbands.

Sale   A temporary reduction in price.

Sample Sale   Sale held at the end of a season to sell overstocks of clothing, as well as that created for promotional purposes. Also called a stock sale.

Sanforized   Trademarked name of a fabric that's been processed to prevent shrinking.

Satin Weave   A weave that produces a subtle sheen and luxurious drape.

Scale   The size of design details and patterns in proportion to the dimensions of the overall garment.

Scotchgard   Trademark for a finish that makes fabrics resistant to grease and water stains.

Seam Finish   A technique used to make a seam edge look neater and/or keep it from raveling.

Seersucker   The quintessential summer suit fabric; a lightweight, usually cotton, fabric with a crinkly striped surface.

Serge   A suiting material characterized by a flat, diagonal rib. The terms *serge* and *twill* are often used synonymously.

Sew-Through Button   One with either two or four holes through which it's secured to the garment.

Shade   The result of adding black to a pure color.

Shank   A short stem, either attached to a button or created with thread, that holds a button away from the fabric. The shank permits the button to fasten easily and sit smoothly.

Shank Button   A button with a little "neck," or shank, with a hole in it on the underside, through which it's sewn to a garment.

Shawl Collar   A collar and lapel that curve seamlessly from the back of the neck down to the front closure.

Sheath   A shaped dress with flattering vertical darts and a curvy silhouette.

Sheer   In hosiery, it refers to the thickness of the yarn. Ultrasheer is the finest and most delicate; opaque, the thickest and most durable.

Shirtwaist   A dress with a bodice styled like a tailored shirt, usually buttoning from the neck to the waist, with either a full or straight skirt.

Shoe Tree   A foot-shaped device inserted into a shoe to help preserve its shape.

Shoulder Pad   Fabric or foam insert used to help strengthen or maintain the shoulder line. Shoulder pads come in many shapes, sizes, and thicknesses.

Silk   A brilliantly lustrous fiber produced by caterpillars.

Single-Needle Stitching   A single needle is used to sew one side of a garment at a time. Double-needle stitching, though faster, is more likely to produce puckered seams.

Sling Back   Any shoe with an open back and a strap around the heel of the foot to hold it in place.

Spandex   A strong fiber that adds stretch and holding power to fabrics, even if only a small percentage is used. Lycra is the trademark for spandex made by DuPont.

Spectator   A two-toned shoe.

Split Leather   The underneath layer of the hide, which is generally thicker and stiffer than top-grain leather.

Sport Jacket   A man's jacket sold without matching trousers. Sport jackets are usually sportier than suit jackets and blazers.

Spread Collar   A widely spread collar.

Straight Collar   Also called the point collar, it's the most common collar of all. The length of the points vary and point downward.

Suede   Leather finished by buffing to produce a velvetlike napped surface. Suede is softer, thinner, and therefore not as durable as regular leather.

Superfine Wool   The finest classification of wool, it's comparable to cashmere. Superfine wool, the finest of which is graded Super 100, comes from strains of Merino sheep.

Suspenders   Adjustable strips or bands of fabric attached to the waistband and worn over the shoulders to hold up trousers.

Tab Collar   Features two small tabs that prop up a tie and hold it securely in place. The tabs are hidden from view once the tie is tied.

Tail   The narrow end of a tie.

Tartan   A plaid of Scottish origin, formed when the threads that run lengthwise are arranged in precisely the same pattern as those that run widthwise, thus producing a balanced design. Think kilt, and you'll get the idea.

Tattersall   A pattern of narrow dark lines crossed to form squares on a white or contrasting colored ground.

Teflon   A fabric finish that helps repel spills and stains.

Telescoping Handles   Handles that pull out and then disappear back into a suitcase.

Tencel   Trademark for a soft, natural fiber made from trees grown on managed tree farms.

Texture   The visual or tactile surface appearance of fabric.

Thrift Shop   A store that sells used clothing.

Tie Coat   Can be single- or double-breasted, with exposed or covered buttons. The latter style, known as a fly front, has the edge on keeping you warmer, since it shields the coat opening from direct contact with the outside.

Tint   The result of adding white to a pure color.

Tone   The result of adding gray to a pure color.

Top-Grain Leather   The leather that is derived from the top layer of the hide and possesses its natural grain. A strong and durable leather.

Trench Coat   A long, water-repellent cloth coat made in a double-breasted style with epaulets, loose shoulder yoke, slotted pockets, and buckled belt. Originally designed for military use in the trenches of World War I.

Triacetate   A synthetic fiber that's related to acetate. Its ability to tolerate heat means that it can be ironed at high temperatures.

Tricot   Knits that exhibit fine ribs on the front, crosswise rows on the back. They have a soft, draping quality.

Tricotene   A fabric with a distinct double twill line used for suits and sportswear.

Tropical Suiting   Lightweight, soft, fluid, usually wool fabrics that provide year-round wear. Think of them as lightweight wools.

Tunic   A thigh-length pullover that usually falls straight from the shoulder.

Turtleneck   A pullover sweater with a very high rib-knit collar that folds over.

Tweed   A general term for rough fabrics woven from wool in a variety of effects, including checks, plaids, flecks, and solids. Because of the coarseness, tweeds are usually saved for lined jackets and trousers. Harris Tweed refers to woolen fabric handwoven on the islands of the Outer Hebrides off the northern coast of Scotland—including the Island of Harris.

Twill Weave   A very durable weave that's characterized by the diagonal ribs that form on one or both sides of the fabric.

Twinset   A cardigan and matching pullover worn together.

Value   A term that refers to the lightness or darkness of a color.

Vamp   The part of the shoe that covers the top of the foot.

Velvet   A tightly woven fabric with a short, dense pile or fuzzy finish, which produces a soft, rich texture. Velveteen has a shorter, less-luxurious pile.

Vicuña   The finest of all animal fibers, vicuña is soft, strong, and expensive to produce—it takes a dozen vicuñas, a small animal of the llama family, to make one piece of cloth.

Virgin Wool   Wool being used for the first time.

Viyella   Trade name for a soft, warm, hard-wearing fabric of 55 percent wool and 45 percent cotton.

Warm Colors   Those with yellow undertones.

Water Repellent   Fabric or material that sheds water easily, usually as a result of tight weaves and chemical treatments.

Waterproof   Fabric or material guaranteed not to absorb water. It's usually made of plastic or vinyl or impregnated with a resin.

Wearing Ease   The extra room built into a garment to permit the wearer to sit, walk, reach, and bend. Ideally, there will be 3 inches of wearing ease in the chest/bust, $3/4$ of an inch at the waist, and 2 inches at the hips.

Windowpane Plaid   Widely spaced stripes that resemble a multipaned window.

Windsor Knot   An oversized knot, the thickest of the three used to tie a tie. It's named for the duke of Windsor, who wore it to complement his wide, spread collars.

Wingtip   Shoe with appliqued leather on the toe, shaped like a bird's spread wings.

Wool   Fiber or fabric derived from the fleece of sheep.

Worsted Wool   Wool that's made up of the harder, smoother, longer, and stronger yarns, it imparts a smooth, crisp look and feel to fabric; woolen yarns—those fashioned of shorter, twisted yarns—are more pliable, less expensive, and create fuzzier fabrics.

Index

331

Q

When You're **Smart** Enough to **Know** That **You** Don't Know It All!

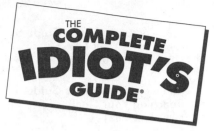

*For all the ups and downs you're sure to encounter in life,
The Complete Idiot's Guides give you
down-to-earth answers and practical solutions.*

Personal Business

The Complete Idiot's Guide to Assertiveness
ISBN: 0-02-861964-1
$16.95

The Complete Idiot's Guide to Business Management
ISBN: 0-02-861744-4
$16.95

The Complete Idiot's Guide to New Product Development
ISBN: 0-02-861952-8
$16.95

The Complete Idiot's Guide to Dynamic Selling
ISBN: 0-02-861952-8
$16.95

The Complete Idiot's Guide to Getting Along with Difficult People
ISBN: 0-02-861597-2
$16.95

The Complete Idiot's Guide to Great Customer Service
ISBN: 0-02-861953-6
$16.95

The Complete Idiot's Guide to Leadership
ISBN: 0-02-861946-3
$16.95

The Complete Idiot's Guide to Marketing Basics
ISBN: 0-02-861490-9
$16.95

The Complete Idiot's Guide to Office Politics
ISBN: 0-02-862397-5
$16.95

The Complete Idiot's Guide to Project Management
ISBN: 0-02-861745-2
$16.95

The Complete Idiot's Guide to Starting a Home Based Business
ISBN: 0-02-861539-5
$16.95

The Complete Idiot's Guide to Successful Business Presentations
ISBN: 0-02-861748-7
$16.95

The Complete Idiot's Guide to Freelancing
ISBN: 0-02-862119-0
$16.95

The Complete Idiot's Guide to Changing Careers
ISBN: 0-02-861977-3
$17.95

The Complete Idiot's Guide to Terrific Business Writing
ISBN: 0-02-861097-0
$16.95

The Complete Idiot's Guide to Getting the Job You Want
ISBN: 1-56761-608-9
$24.95

The Complete Idiot's Guide to Managing Your Time
ISBN: 0-02-861039-3
$14.95

The Complete Idiot's Guide to Speaking in Public With Confidence
ISBN: 0-02-861038-5
$16.95

The Com5plete Idiot's Guide to Winning Through Negotiation
ISBN: 0-02-861037-7
$16.95

The Complete Idiot's Guide to Managing People
ISBN: 0-02-861036-9
$18.95

The Complete Idiot's Guide to a Great Retirement
ISBN: 0-02-861036-9
$16.95

The Complete Idiot's Guide to Starting Your Own Business
ISBN: 1-56761-529-5
$16.99

The Complete Idiot's Guide to Protecting Yourself from Everyday Legal Hassles
ISBN: 1-56761-602-X
$16.99

The Complete Idiot's Guide to Surviving Divorce
ISBN: 0-02-861101-3
$16.95

The Complete Idiot's Guide to
Organizing Your Life
ISBN: 0-02-861090-3
$16.95

The Complete Idiot's Guide to
Reaching Your Goals
ISBN: 0-02-862114-X
$16.95

The Complete Idiot's Guide to
the Perfect Cover Letter
ISBN: 0-02-861960-9
$14.95

The Complete Idiot's Guide to
the Perfect Interview
ISBN: 0-02-861945-5
$14.95

The Complete Idiot's Guide to
the Perfect Resume
ISBN: 0-02-861093-8
$16.95

Personal Finance

The Complete Idiot's Guide to
Buying Insurance and Annu-
ities
ISBN: 0-02-861113-6
$16.95

The Complete Idiot's Guide to
Managing Your Money
ISBN: 1-56761-530-9
$16.95

The Complete Idiot's Guide to
Making Money with Mutual
Funds
ISBN: 1-56761-637-2
$16.95

The Complete Idiot's Guide to
Buying and Selling a Home
ISBN: 0-02-861959-5
$16.95

The Complete Idiot's Guide to
Getting Rich
ISBN: 1-56761-509-0
$16.95

The Complete Idiot's Guide to
Finance and Accounting
ISBN: 0-02-861752-5
$16.95

The Complete Idiot's Guide to
Investing Like a Pro
ISBN:0-02-862044-5
$16.95

The Complete Idiot's Guide to
Making Money After You
Retire
ISBN:0-02-862410-6
$16.95

The Complete Idiot's Guide to
Making Money on Wall Street
ISBN:0-02-861958-7
$16.95

The Complete Idiot's Guide to
Personal Finance in Your 20s
and 30s
ISBN:0-02-862415-7
$16.95

The Complete Idiot's Guide to
Wills and Estates
ISBN: 0-02-861747-9
$16.95

The Complete Idiot's Guide to
401(k) Plans
ISBN: 0-02-861948-X
$16.95

Lifestyle

The Complete Idiot's Guide to
Etiquette
ISBN0-02-861094-6
$16.95

The Complete Idiot's Guide to
Dating
ISBN: 0-02-861052-0
$14.95

The Complete Idiot's Guide to
Trouble-Free Car Care
ISBN: 0-02-861041-5
$16.95

The Complete Idiot's Guide to
the Perfect Wedding
ISBN: 0-02-861963-3
$16.95

The Complete Idiot's Guide to
the Perfect Vacation
ISBN: 1-56761-531-7
$14.99

The Complete Idiot's Guide to
Trouble-Free Home Repair
ISBN: 0-02-861042-3
$16.95

The Complete Idiot's Guide to
Getting Into College
ISBN: 1-56761-508-2
$14.95

The Complete Idiot's Guide to
a Healthy Relationship
ISBN: 0-02-861087-3
$17.95

The Complete Idiot's Guide to
Dealing with In-Laws
ISBN: 0-02-862107-7
$16.95

The Complete Idiot's Guide to
Choosing, Training, and
Raising a Dog
ISBN: 0-02-861098-9
$16.95

The Complete Idiot's Guide to
Fun and Tricks with Your Dog
ISBN: 0-87605-083-6
$14.95

The Complete Idiot's Guide to
Living with a Cat
ISBN: 0-02-861278-7
$16.95

The Complete Idiot's Guide to
Turtles and Tortoises
ISBN: 0-87605-143-3
$16.95

Leisure/Hobbies

The Complete Idiot's Guide to
Baking
ISBN: 0-02-861954-4
$16.95

The Complete Idiot's Guide to
Beer
ISBN: 0-02-861717-7
$16.95

The Complete Idiot's Guide to
Cooking Basics
ISBN: 0-02-861974-9
$18.95

The Complete Idiot's Guide to
Entertaining
ISBN: 0-02-861095-4
$16.95

The Complete Idiot's Guide to
Mixing Drinks
ISBN: 0-02-861941-2
$16.95

The Complete Idiot's Guide to
Wine
ISBN: 0-02-861273-6
$16.95

The Complete Idiot's Guide to
Antiques and Collectibles
ISBN: 0-02-861595-6
$16.95

The Complete Idiot's Guide to
Boating and Sailing
ISBN: 0-02-862124-7
$18.95

The Complete Idiot's Guide to
Bridge
ISBN: 0-02-861735-5
$16.95

The Complete Idiot's Guide to
Chess
ISBN: 0-02-861736-3
$16.95

The Complete Idiot's Guide to
Cigars
ISBN: 0-02-861975-7
$17.95

The Complete Idiot's Guide to
Crafts with Kids
ISBN: 0-02-862406-8
$16.95

The Complete Idiot's Guide to
Fishing Basics
ISBN: 0-02-861598-0
$16.95

The Complete Idiot's Guide to
Gambling Like a Pro
ISBN: 0-02-861102-0
$16.95

The Complete Idiot's Guide to
Hiking and Camping
ISBN: 0-02-861100-4
$16.95

The Complete Idiot's Guide to
Needlecrafts
ISBN: 0-02-862123-9
$16.95

The Complete Idiot's Guide to
Photography
ISBN: 0-02-861092-X
$16.95

The Complete Idiot's Guide to
Quilting
ISBN: 0-02-862411-4
$16.95

The Complete Idiot's Guide to
Yoga
ISBN: 0-02-861949-8
$16.95

The Complete Idiot's Guide to
the Beatles
ISBN: 0-02-862130-1
$18.95

The Complete Idiot's Guide to
Elvis
ISBN: 0-02-861873-4
$18.95

The Complete Idiot's Guide to
Understanding Football Like a
Pro
ISBN:0-02-861743-6
$16.95

The Complete Idiot's Guide to
Golf
ISBN: 0-02-861760-6
$16.95

The Complete Idiot's Guide to
Motorcycles
ISBN: 0-02-862416-5
$17.95

The Complete Idiot's Guide to
Pro Wrestling
ISBN: 0-02-862395-9
$17.95

The Complete Idiot's Guide to
Extra-Terrestrial Intelligence
ISBN: 0-02-862387-8
$16.95

Health and Fitness

The Complete Idiot's Guide to
Managed Health Care
ISBN: 0-02-862165-4
$17.95

The Complete Idiot's Guide to
Getting and Keeping Your
Perfect Body
ISBN: 0-02-861276-0
$16.95

The Complete Idiot's Guide to
First Aid Basics
ISBN: 0-02-861099-7
$16.95

The Complete Idiot's Guide to
Vitamins
ISBN: 0-02-862116-6
$16.95

The Complete Idiot's Guide to
Losing Weight
ISBN: 0-02-862113-1
$17.95

The Complete Idiot's Guide to
Tennis
ISBN: 0-02-861746-0
$18.95

The Complete Idiot's Guide to
Tae Kwon Do
ISBN: 0-02-862389-4
$17.95

The Complete Idiot's Guide to
Breaking Bad Habits
ISBN: 0-02-862110-7
$16.95

The Complete Idiot's Guide to
Healthy Stretching
ISBN: 0-02-862127-1
$16.95

The Complete Idiot's Guide to
Beautiful Skin
ISBN: 0-02-862408-4
$16.95

The Complete Idiot's Guide to
Eating Smart
ISBN: 0-02-861276-0
$16.95

The Complete Idiot's Guide to
First Aid
ISBN: 0-02-861099-7
$16.95

The Complete Idiot's Guide to
Getting a Good Night's Sleep
ISBN: 0-02-862394-0
$16.95

The Complete Idiot's Guide to
a Happy, Healthy Heart
ISBN: 0-02-862393-2
$16.95

The Complete Idiot's Guide to
Stress
ISBN: 0-02-861086-5
$16.95

The Complete Idiot's Guide to
Jogging and Running
ISBN: 0-02-862386-X
$17.95

The Complete Idiot's Guide to
Adoption
ISBN: 0-02-862108-5
$18.95

The Complete Idiot's Guide to
Bringing Up Baby
ISBN: 0-02-861957-9
$16.95

The Complete Idiot's Guide to
Grandparenting
ISBN: 0-02-861976-5
$16.95

The Complete Idiot's Guide to
Parenting a Preschooler and
Toddler
ISBN: 0-02-861733-9
$16.95

The Complete Idiot's Guide to
Raising a Teenager
ISBN: 0-02-861277-9
$16.95

The Complete Idiot's Guide to
Single Parenting
ISBN: 0-02-862409-2
$16.95

The Complete Idiot's Guide to
Stepparenting
ISBN: 0-02-862407-6
$16.95

Education

The Complete Idiot's Guide to
American History
ISBN: 0-02-861275-2
$16.95

The Complete Idiot's Guide to
British Royalty
ISBN: 0-02-862346-0
$18.95

The Complete Idiot's Guide to
Civil War
ISBN: 0-02-862122-0
$16.95

The Complete Idiot's Guide to
Classical Mythology
ISBN: 0-02-862385-1
$16.95

The Complete Idiot's Guide to
Creative Writing
ISBN: 0-02-861734-7
$16.95

The Complete Idiot's Guide to
Dinosaurs
ISBN: 0-02-862390-8
$17.95

The Complete Idiot's Guide to
Genealogy
ISBN: 0-02-861947-1
$16.95

The Complete Idiot's Guide to
Geography
ISBN: 0-02-861955-2
$16.95

The Complete Idiot's Guide to
Getting Published
ISBN: 0-02-862392-4
$16.95

The Complete Idiot's Guide to
Grammar & Style
ISBN: 0-02-861956-0
$16.95

The Complete Idiot's Guide to
an MBA
ISBN: 0-02-862164-4
$17.95

The Complete Idiot's Guide to
Philosophy
ISBN:0-02-861981-1
$16.95

The Complete Idiot's Guide to
Classical Music
ISBN: 0-02-8611634-0
$16.95

The Complete Idiot's Guide to
Learning Spanish On Your
Own
ISBN: 0-02-861040-7
$16.95

The Complete Idiot's Guide to
Learning French on Your Own
ISBN: 0-02-861043-1
$16.95

The Complete Idiot's Guide to
learning German on Your Own
ISBN: 0-02-861962-5
$16.95

The Complete Idiot's Guide to
Learning Italian on Your Own
ISBN: 0-02-862125-5
$16.95

The Complete Idiot's Guide to
Learning Sign Language
ISBN: 0-02-862388-6
$16.95

The Complete Idiot's Guide to
Astrology
ISBN: 0-02-861951-X
$16.95

The Complete Idiot's Guide to
the World's Religions
ISBN: 0-02-861730-4
$16.95

Look for the Complete Idiot's Guides at your local bookseller, or call 1–800–428–5331 for more information.

You can also check us out on the web at
http://www.mcp.com/mgr/idiot

alpha
books